Serenity's Self-Care Routine:
A Girl's Guide to Healthy Habits

Danielle M. Jackson

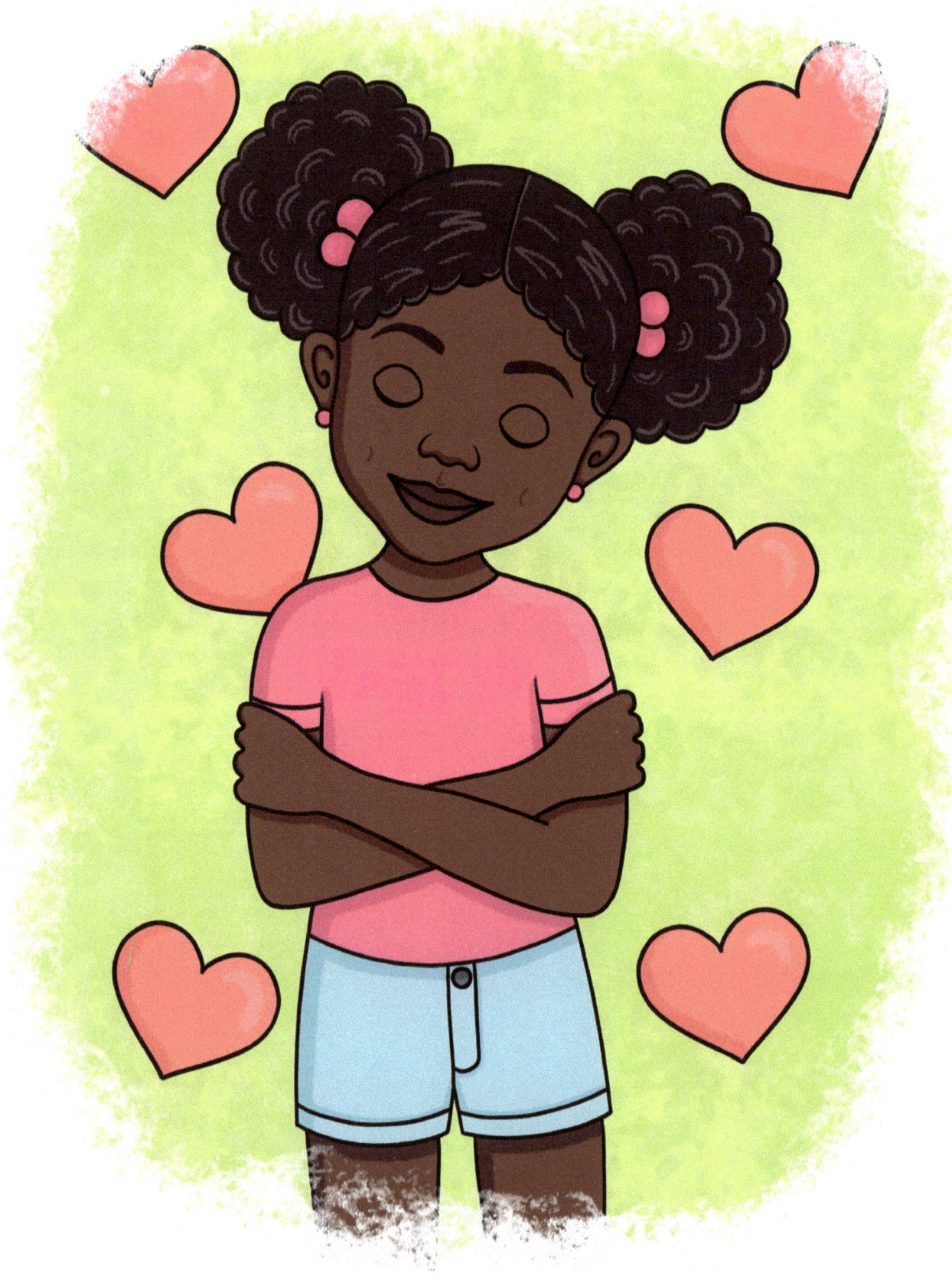

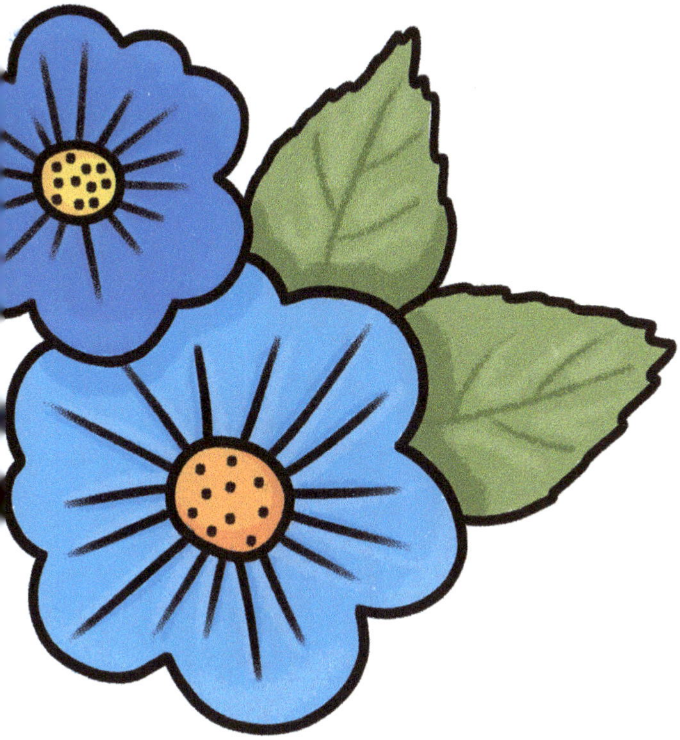

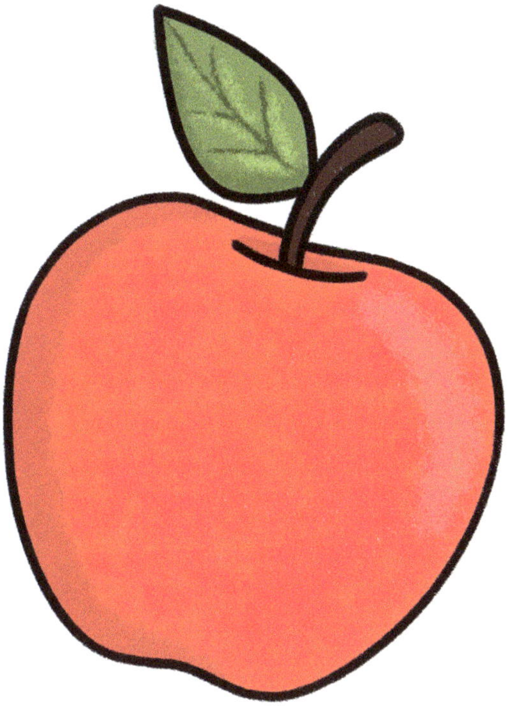

Serenity enjoys her self-care routine. She established this routine because school-life balance allows her to be her best self.

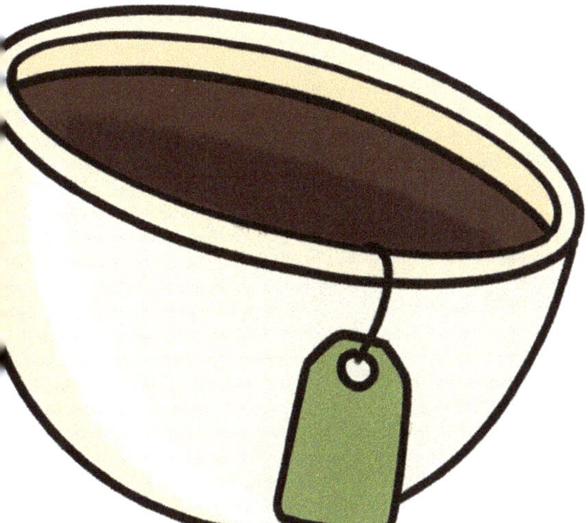

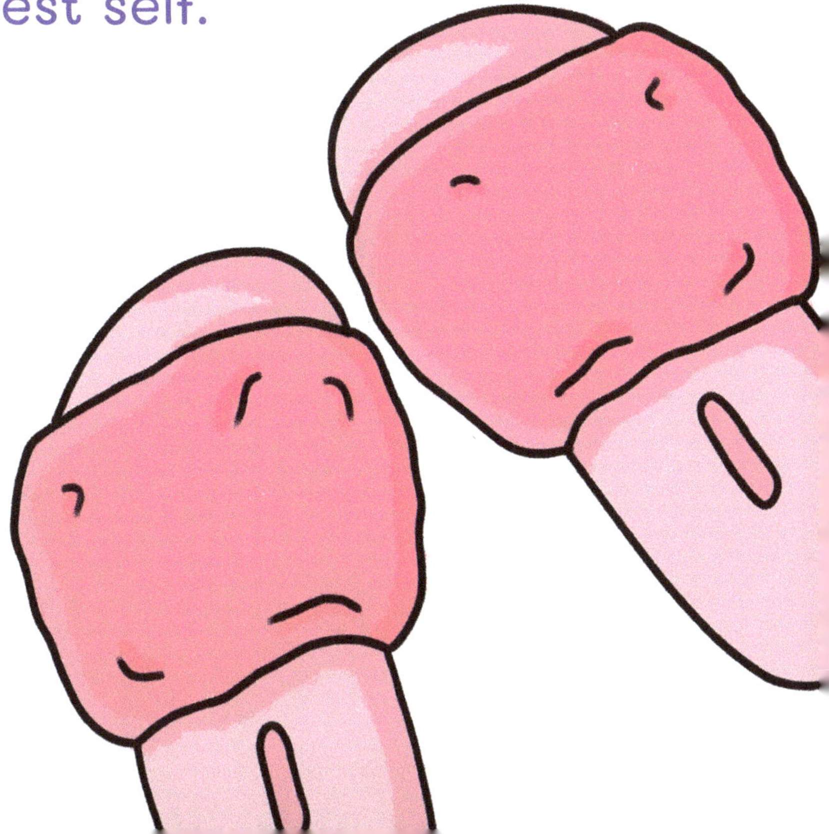

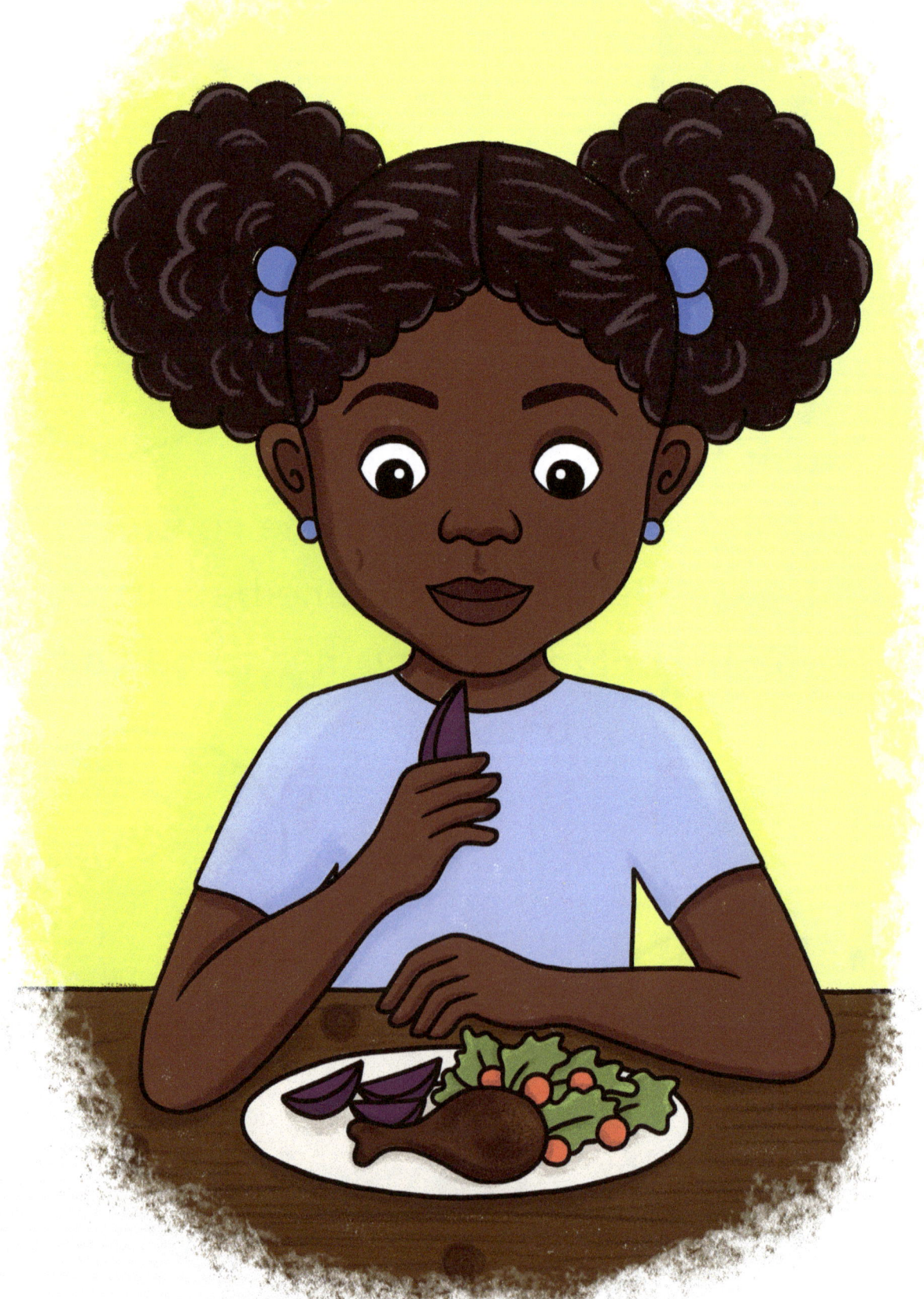

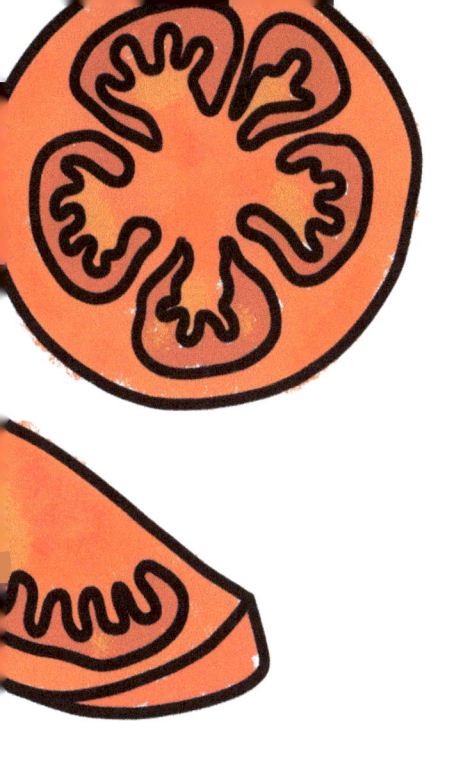
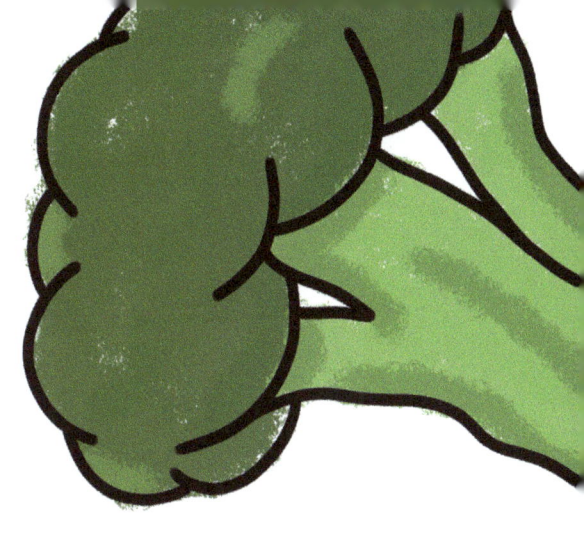

Serenity makes it her business to eat foods that help her body perform well. She appreciates foods that are not only nutritious but delicious.

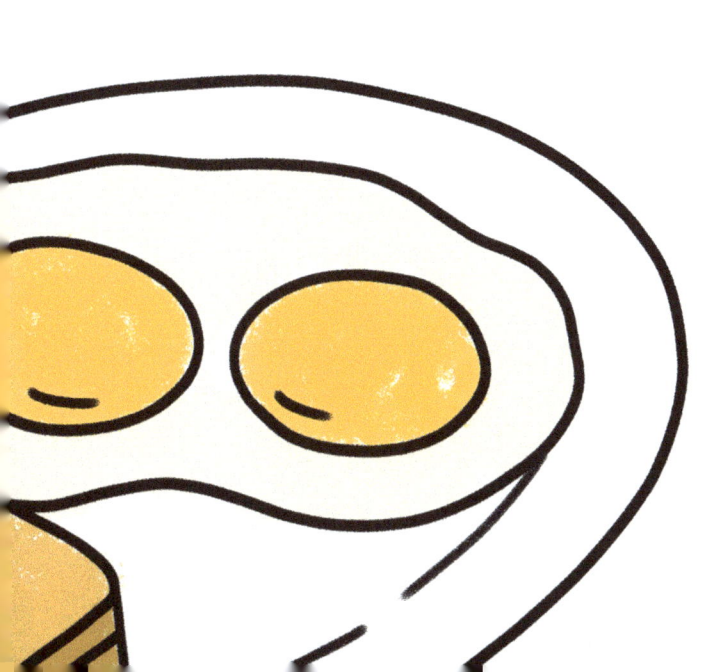
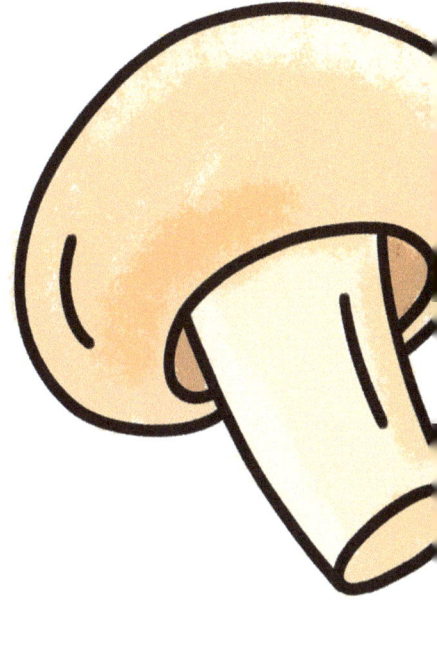

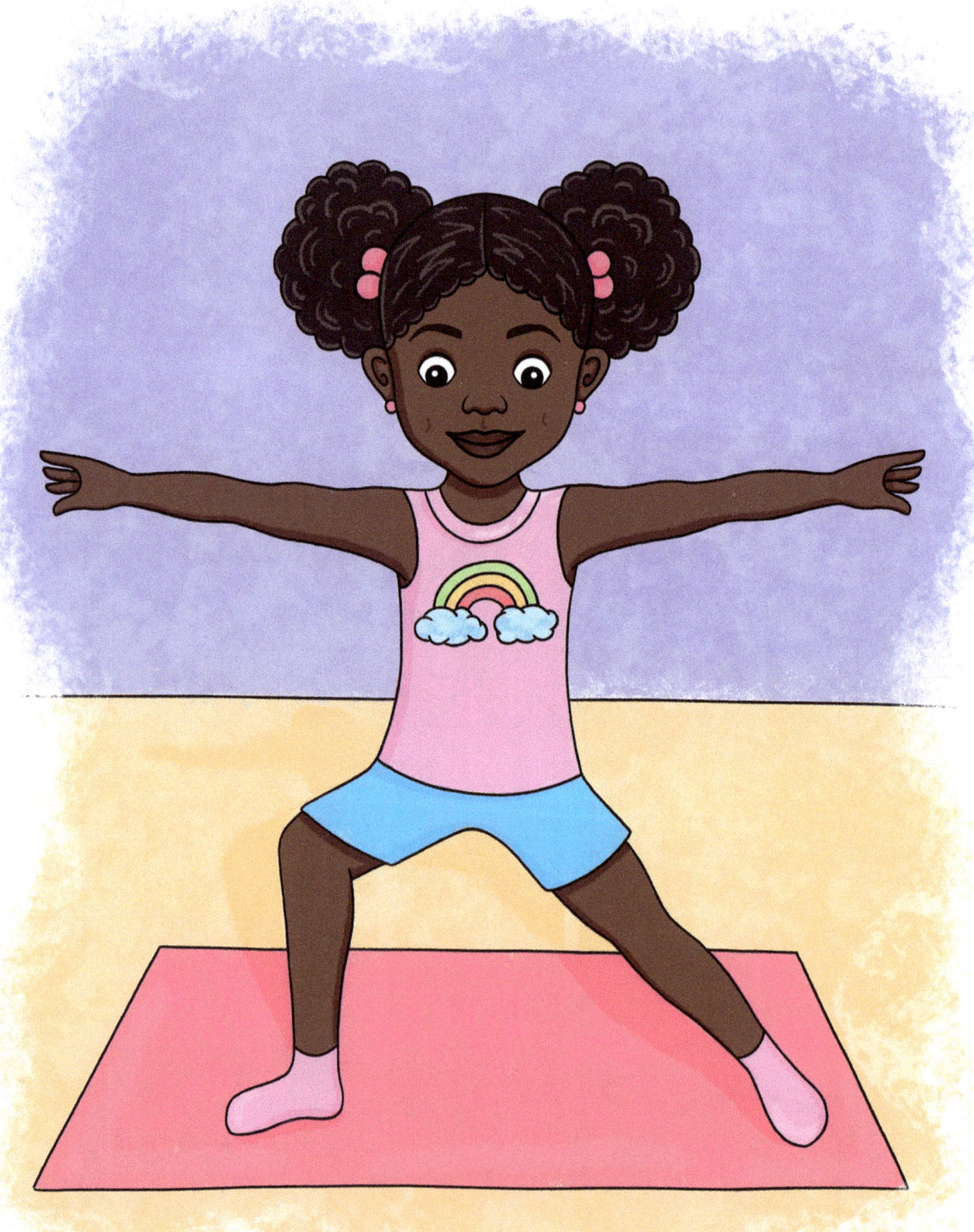

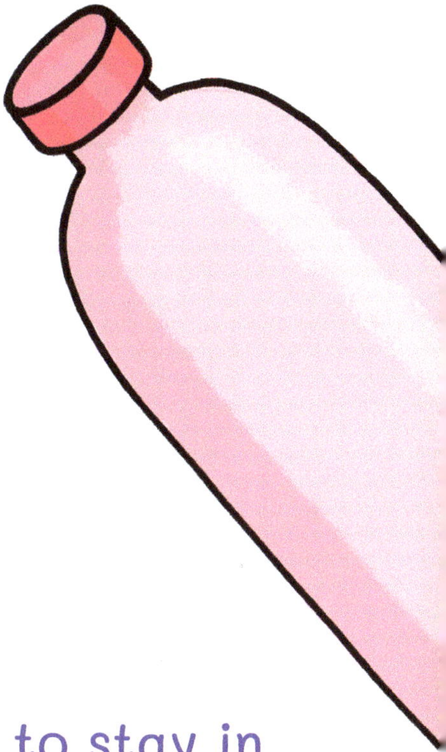

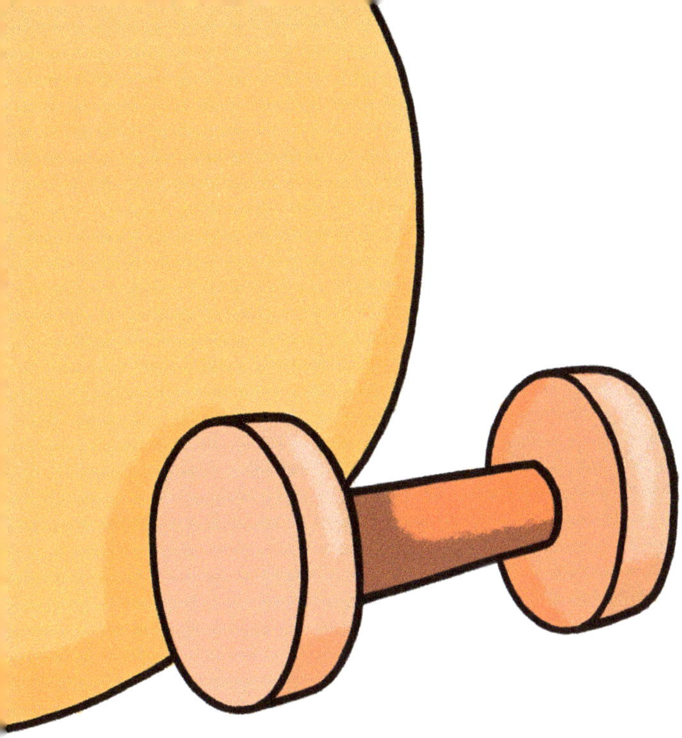

Practicing yoga allows Serenity to stay in tune with her body. Yoga also gives her a personal sense of freedom.

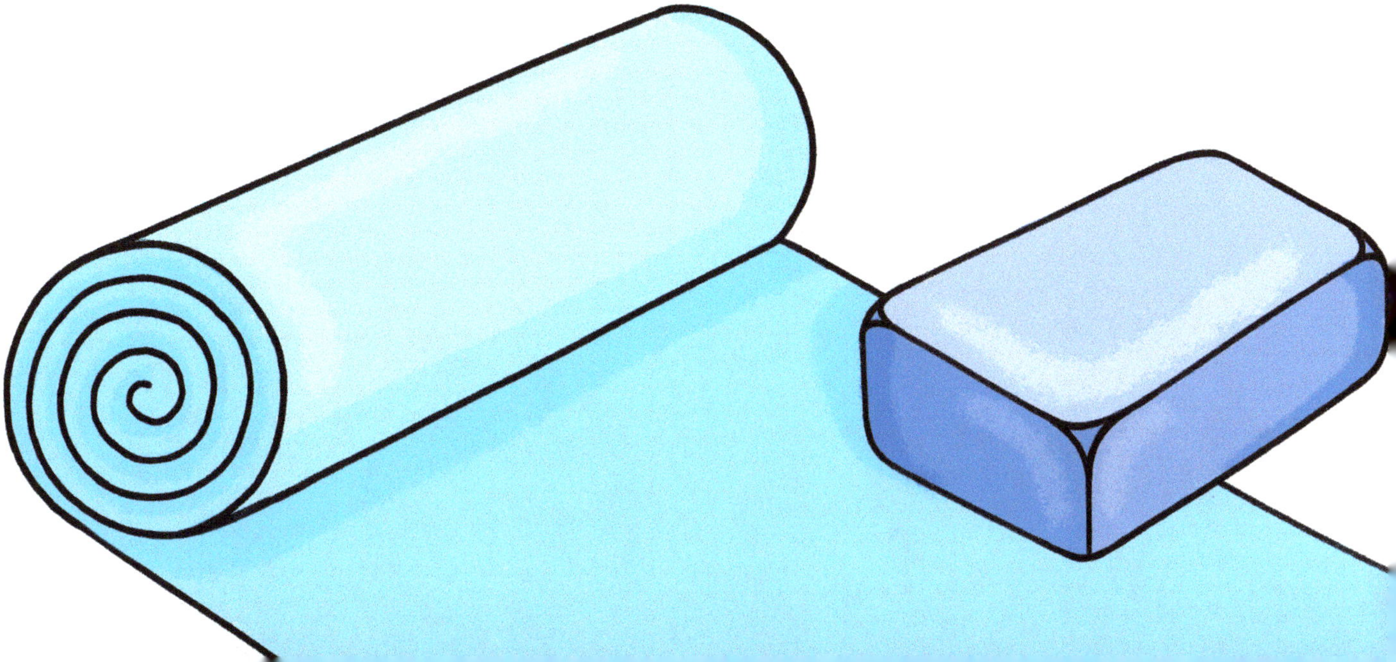

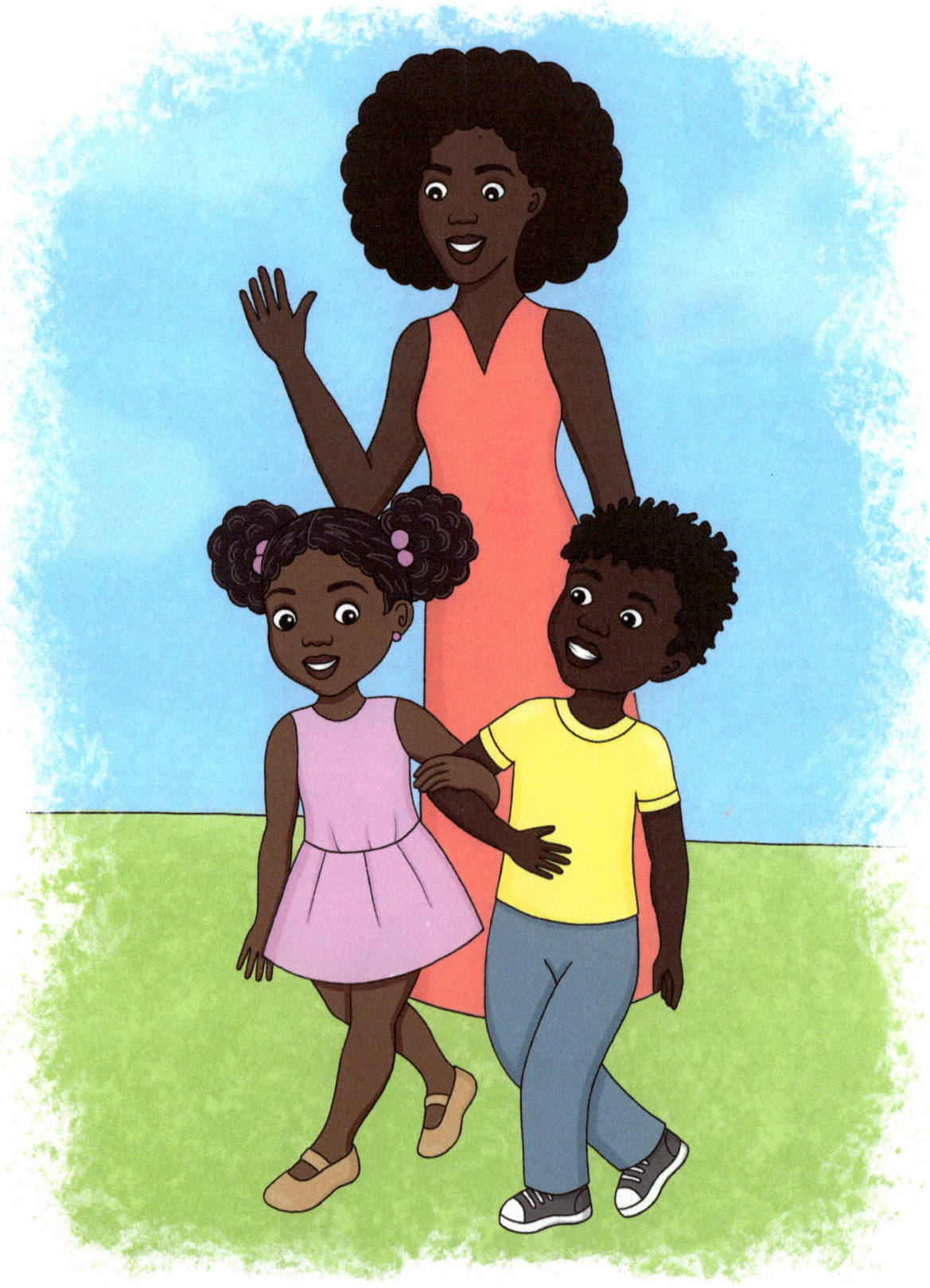

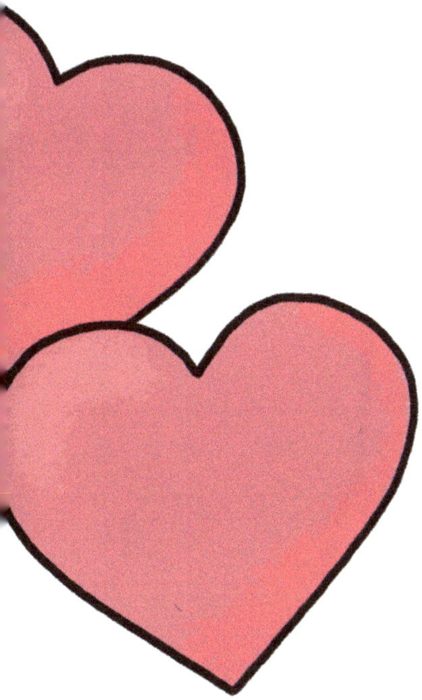

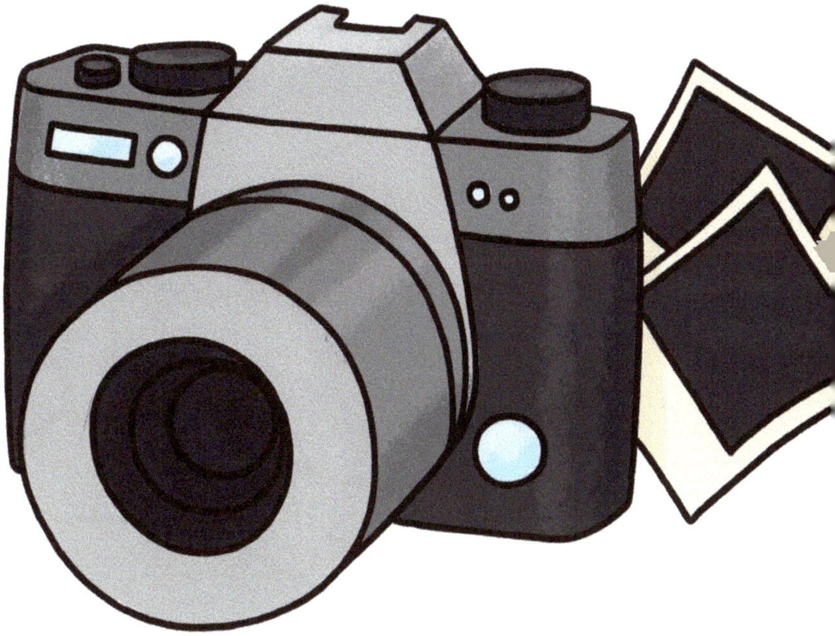

Let the good times begin! Serenity adores her family and friends along with the beautiful memories they create together.

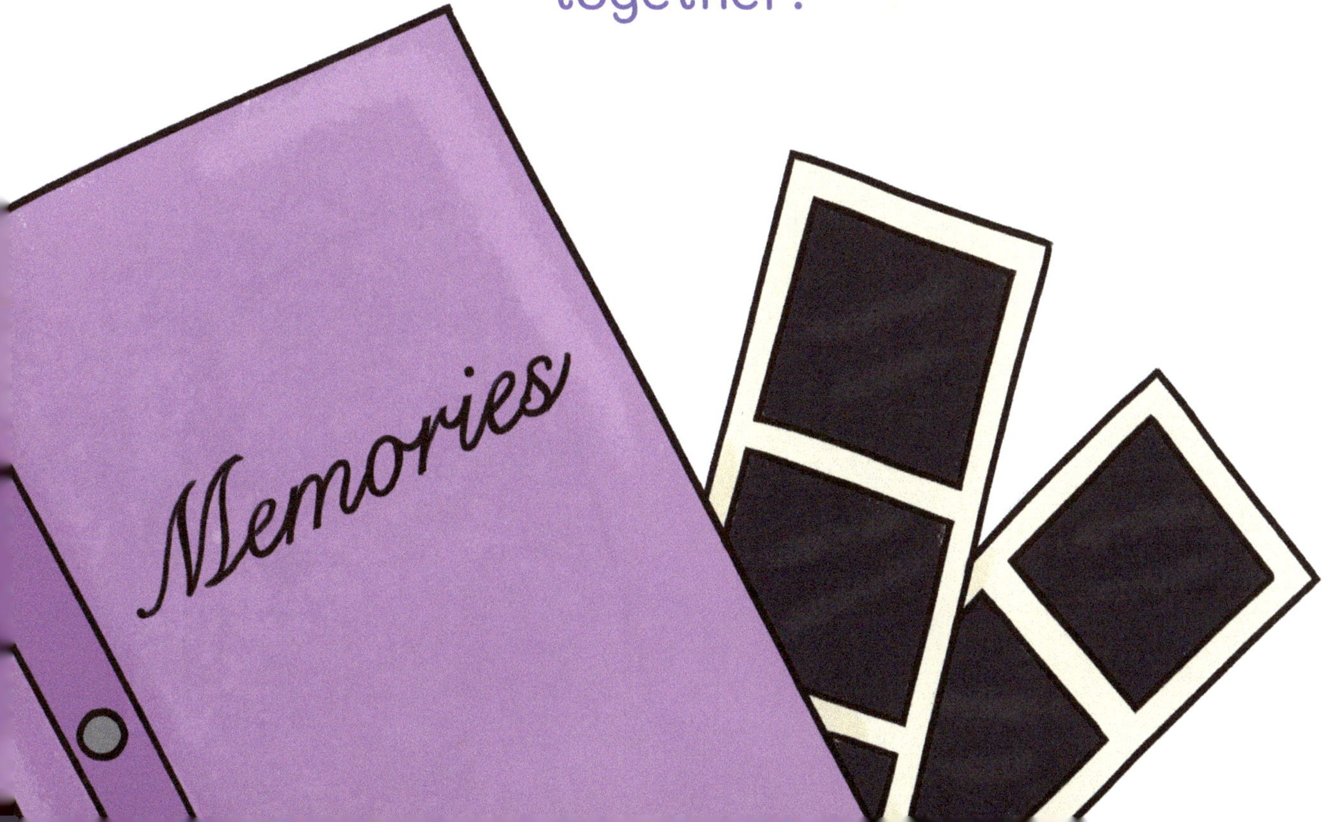

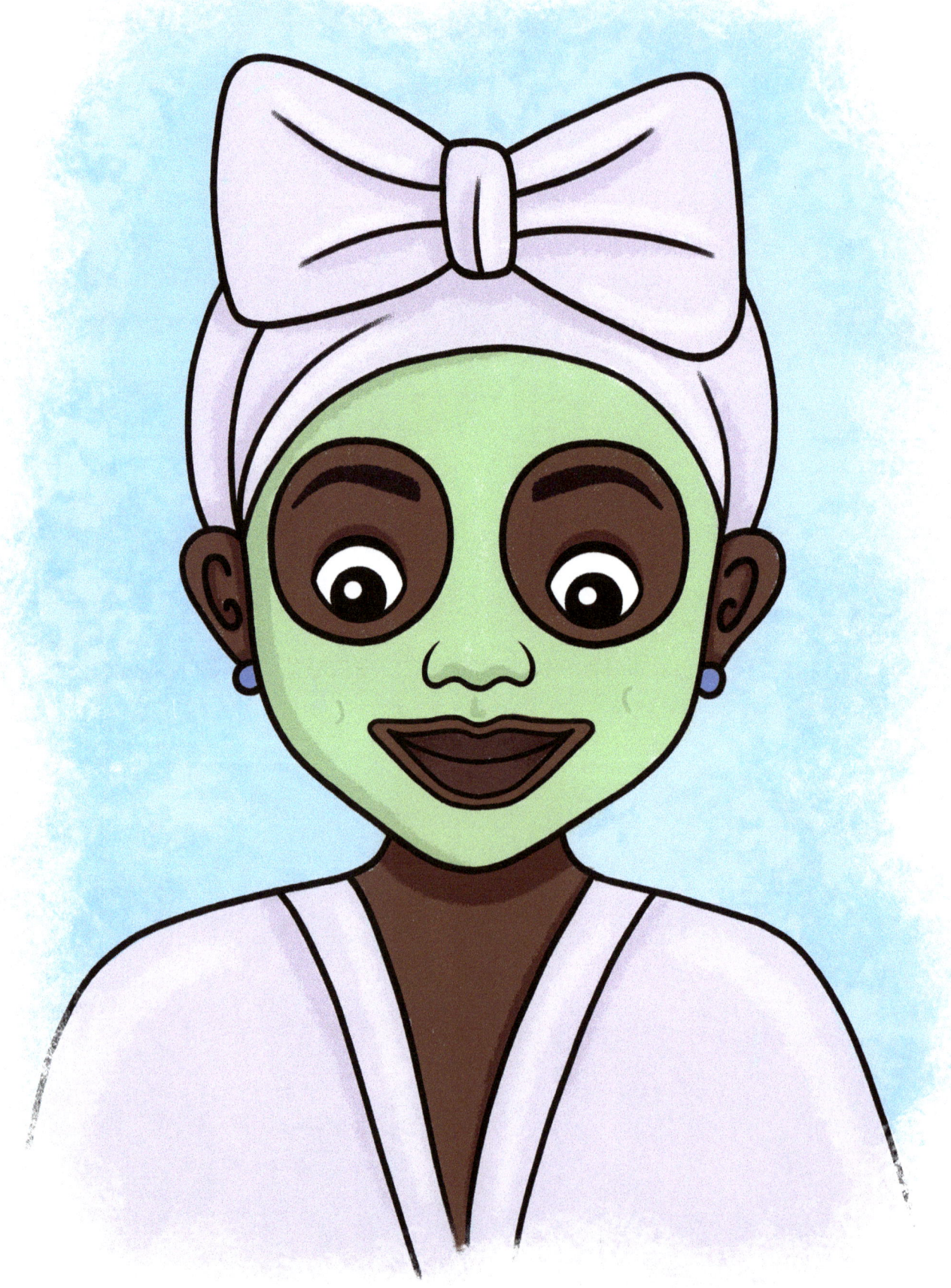

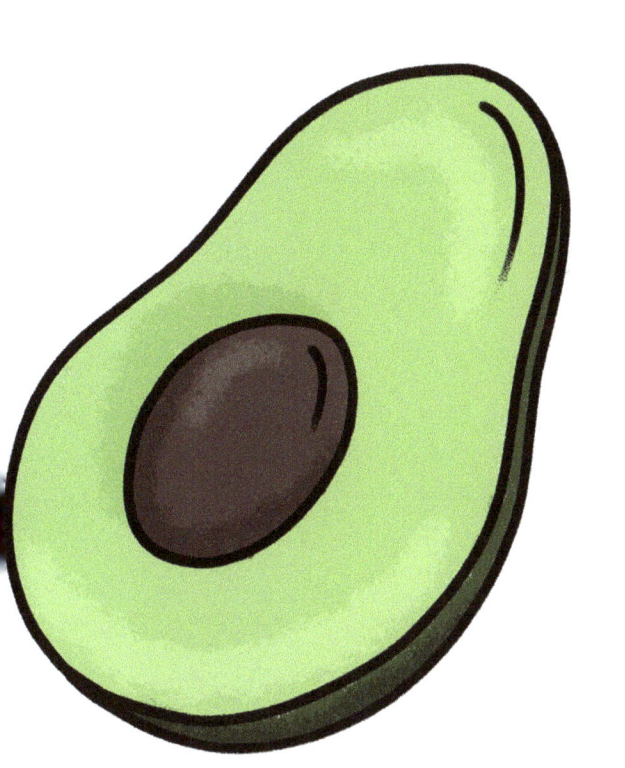
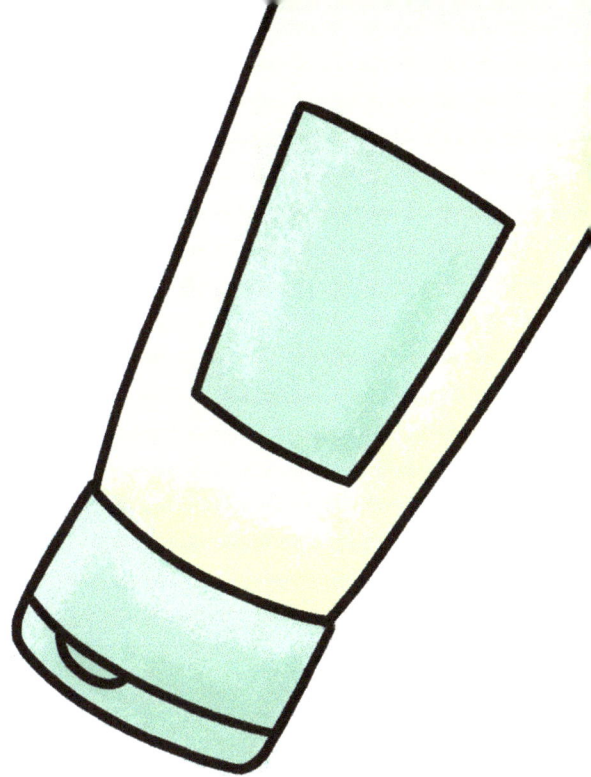

Serenity is very fond of the way her face mask makes her skin glow and feel. Sometimes she adds special ingredients to spice things up!

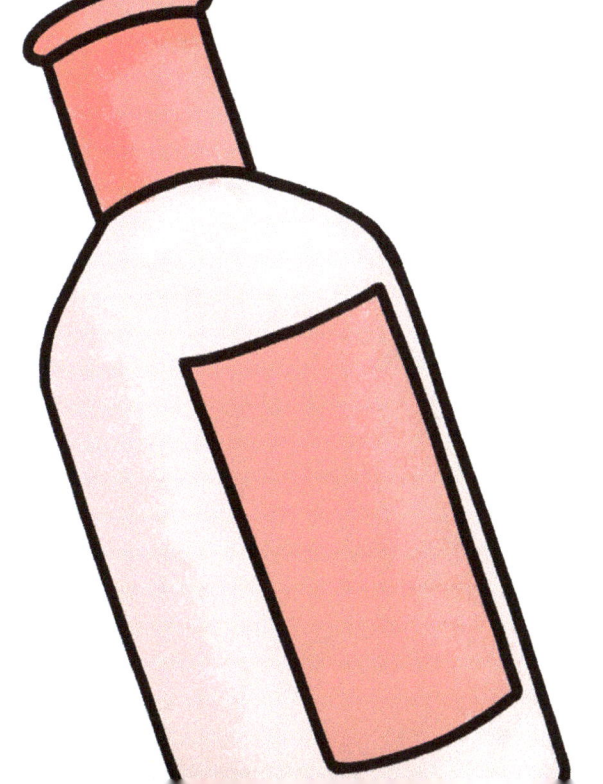
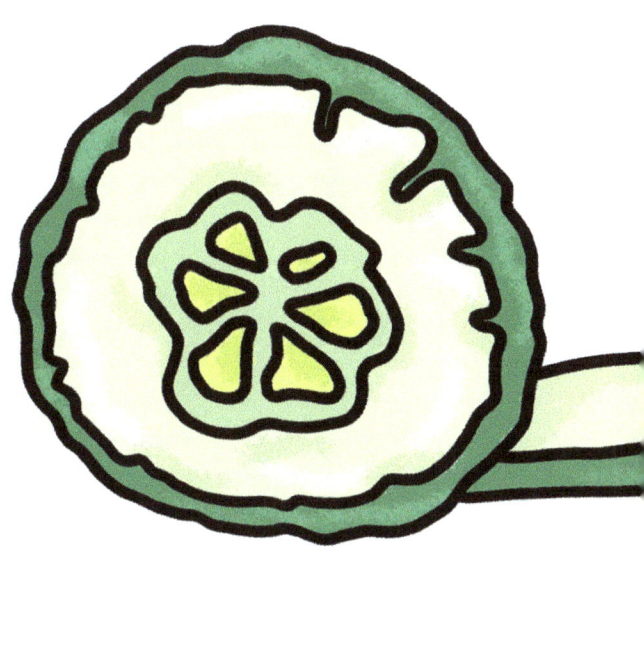

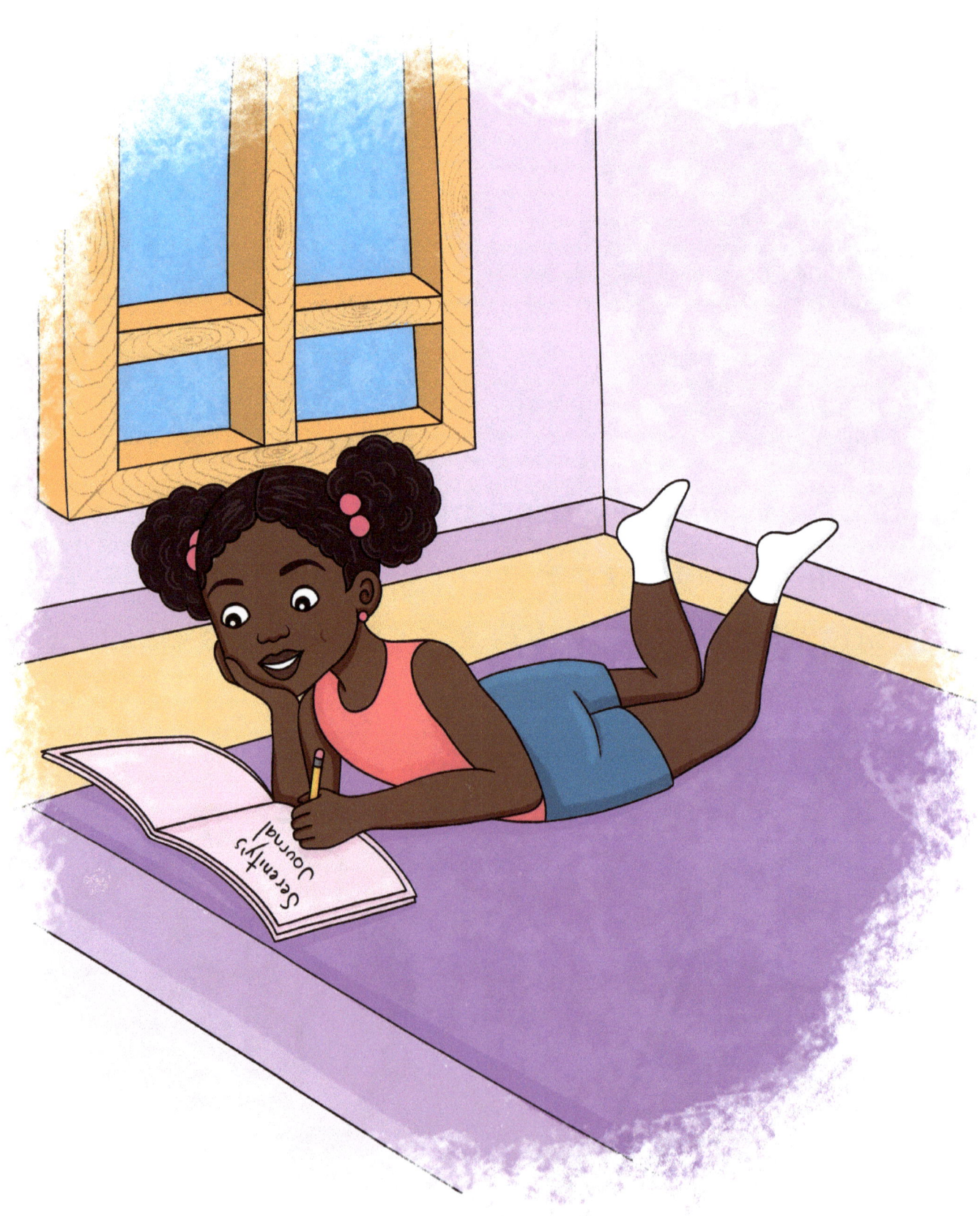

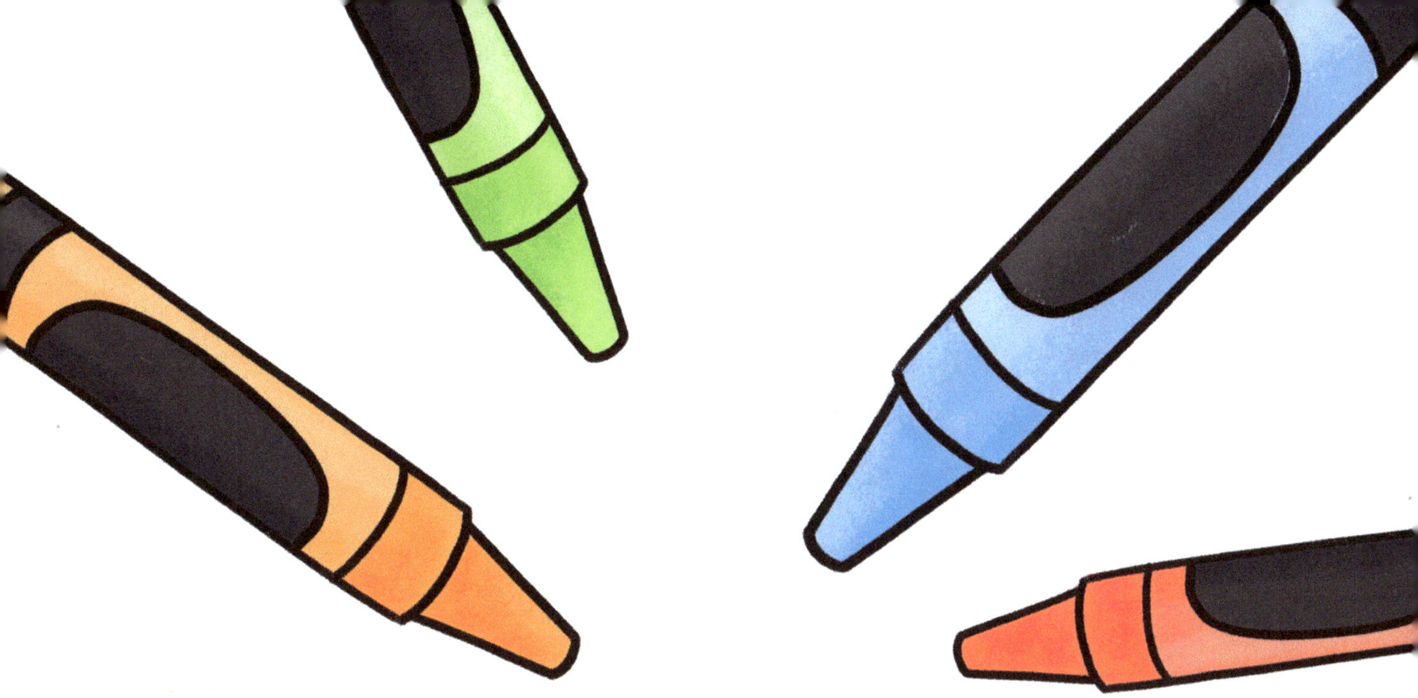

Journaling is Serenity's way of organizing and processing her personal thoughts. By keeping a journal, she is free to express her emotions privately.

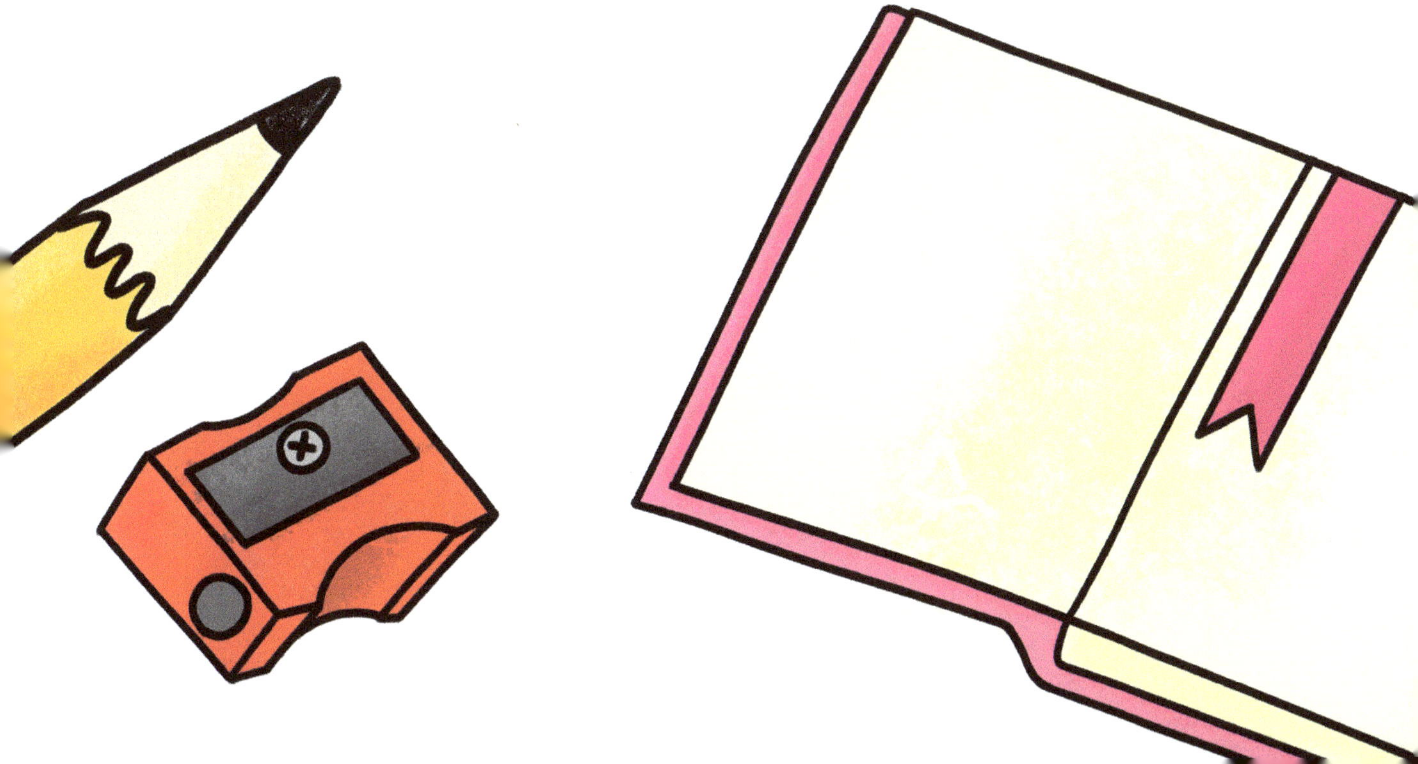

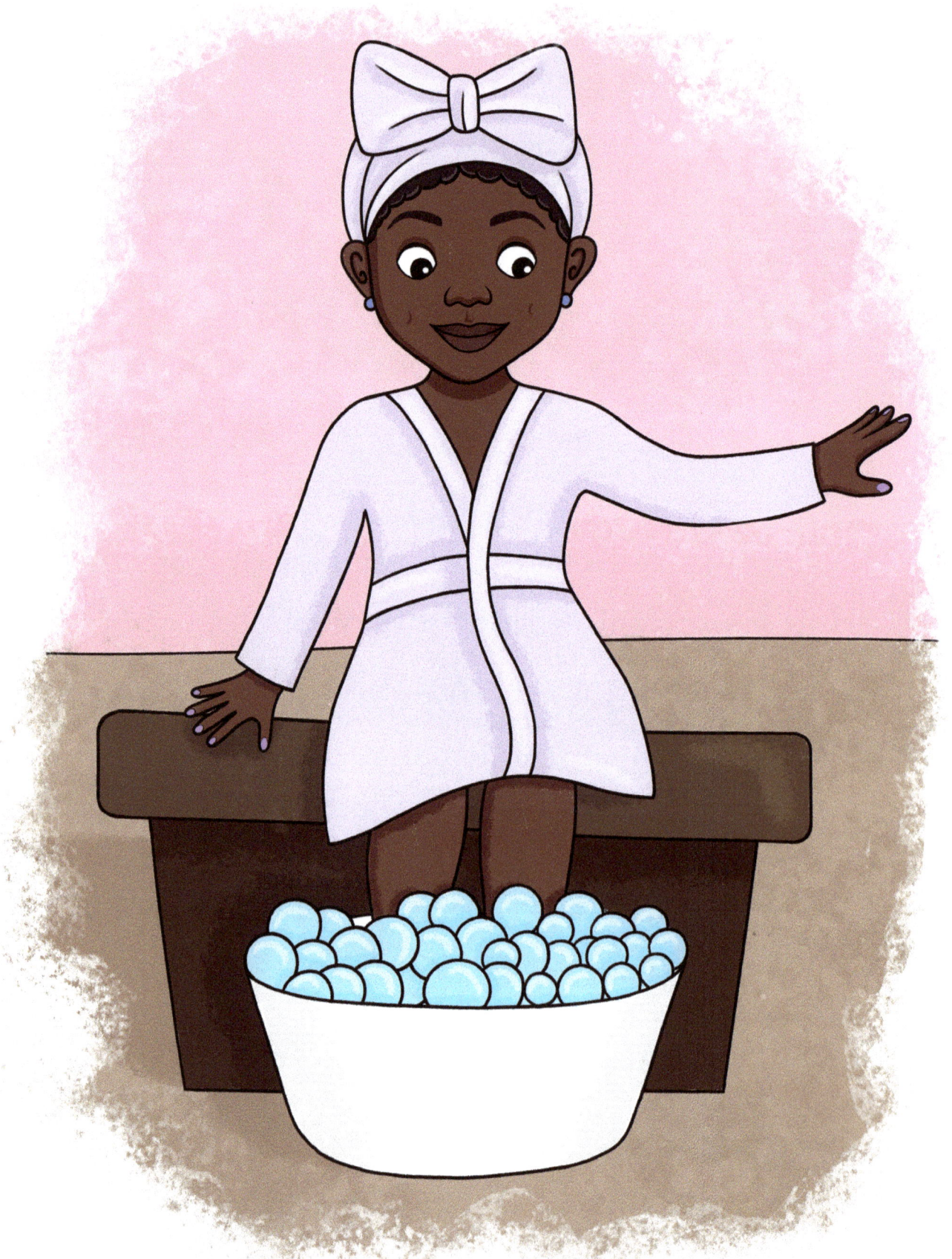

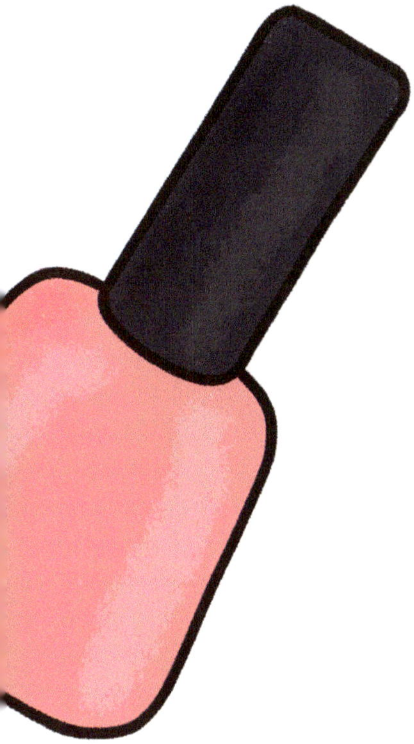

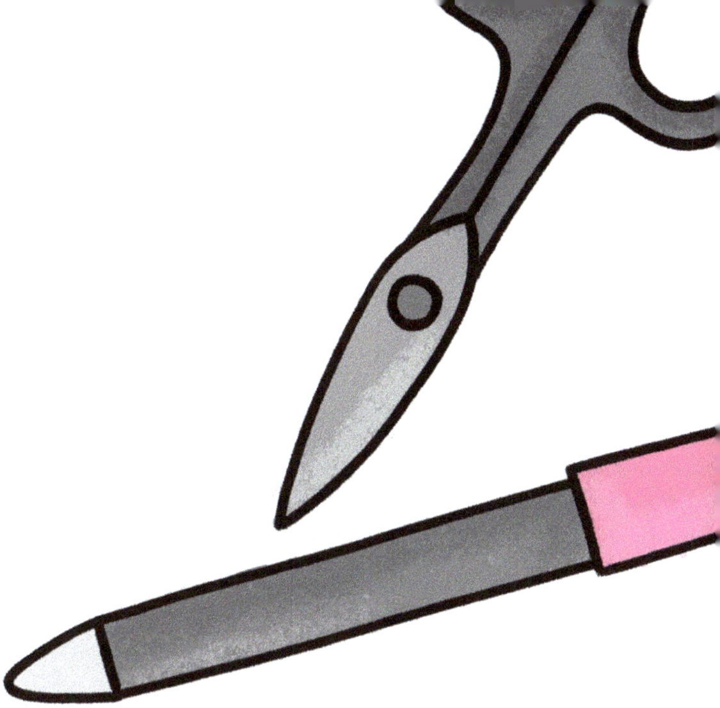

Spa-like treatments make Serenity feel like a princess. She appreciates the bright colors that compliment her unique fashion sense.

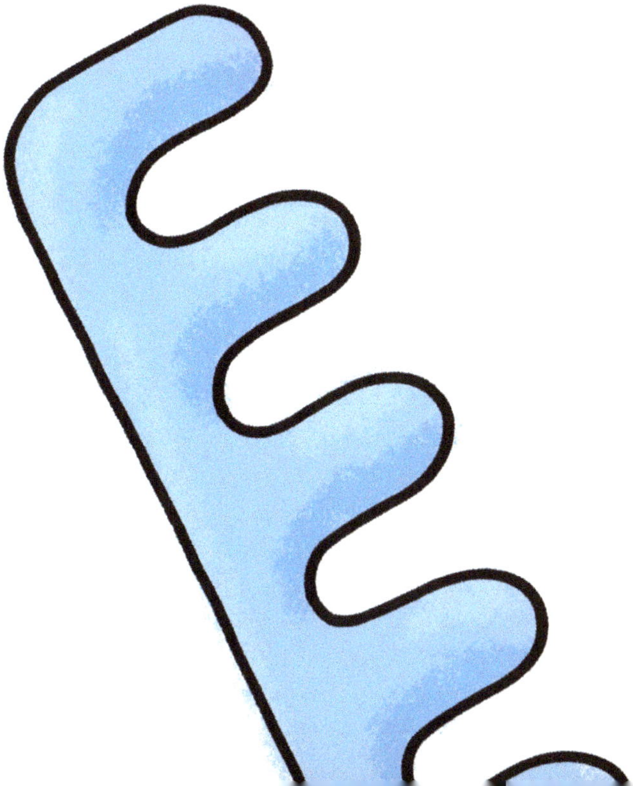

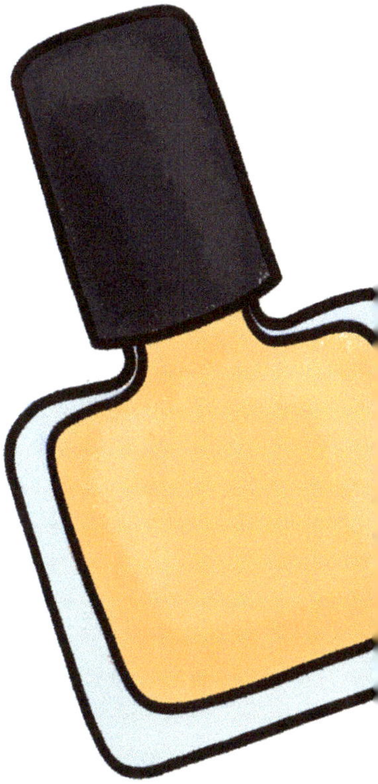

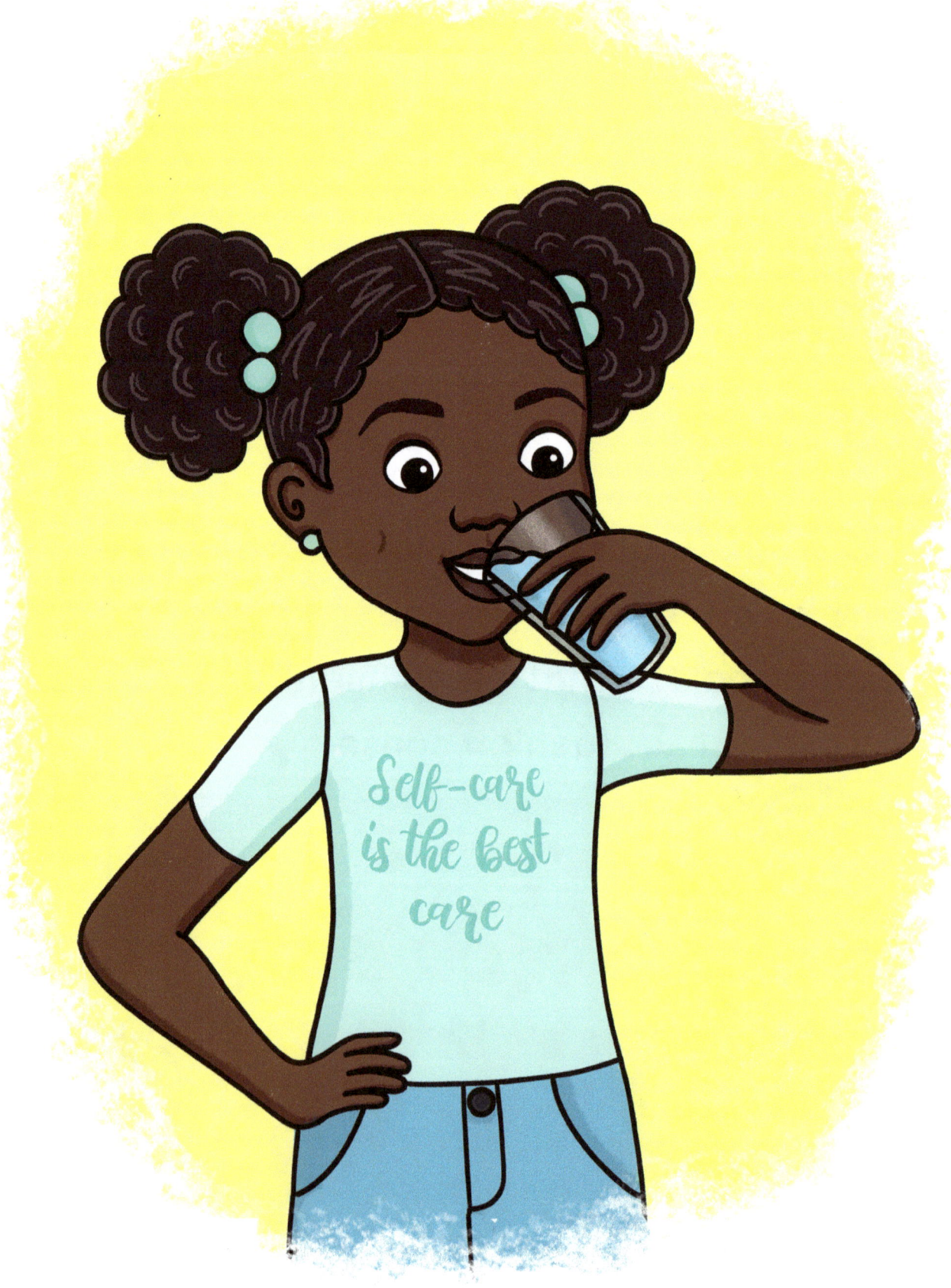

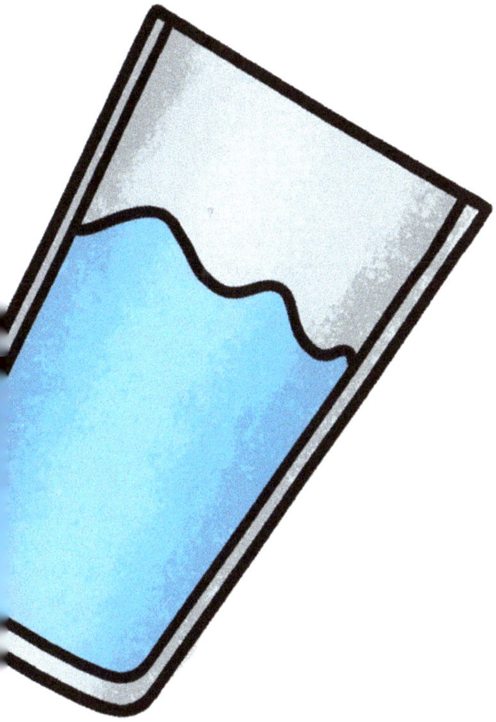

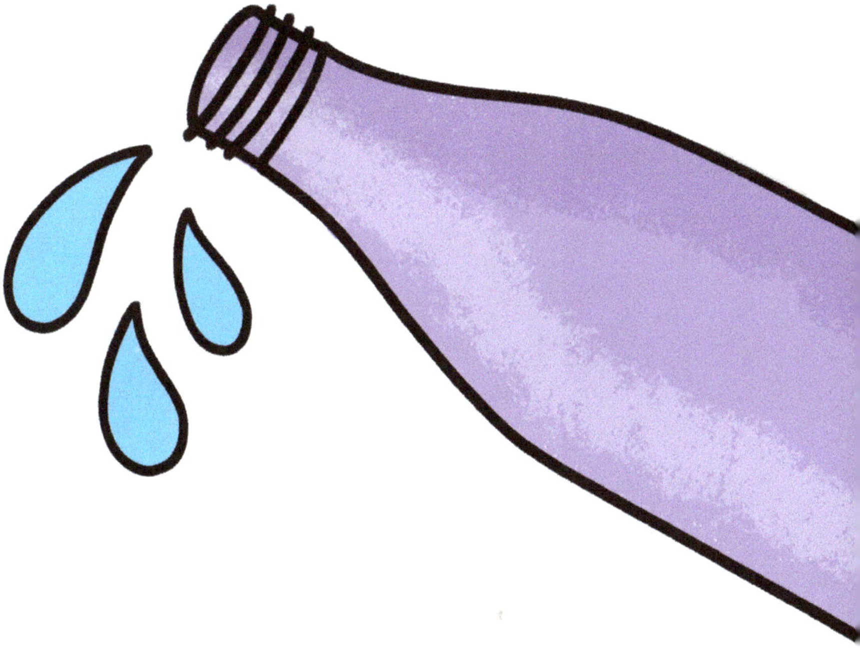

Water is just what the body ordered. Serenity enjoys drinking her fair share of water to quench her thirst and help her body stay hydrated and healthy.

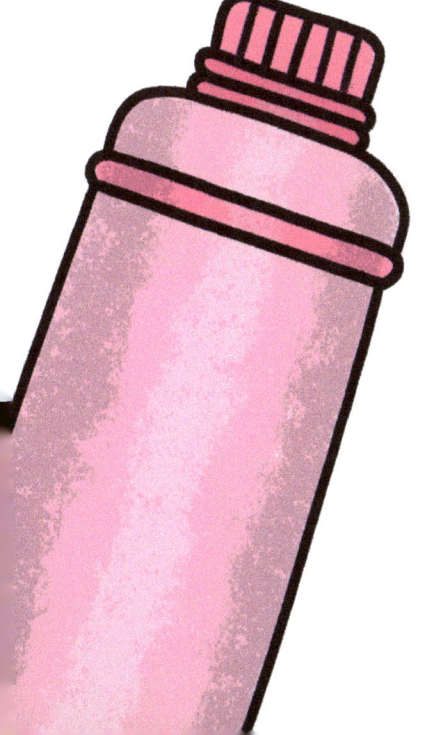
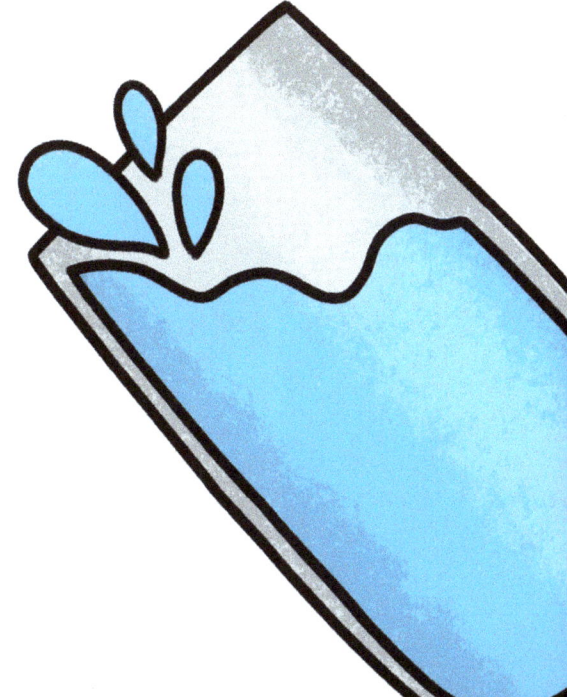

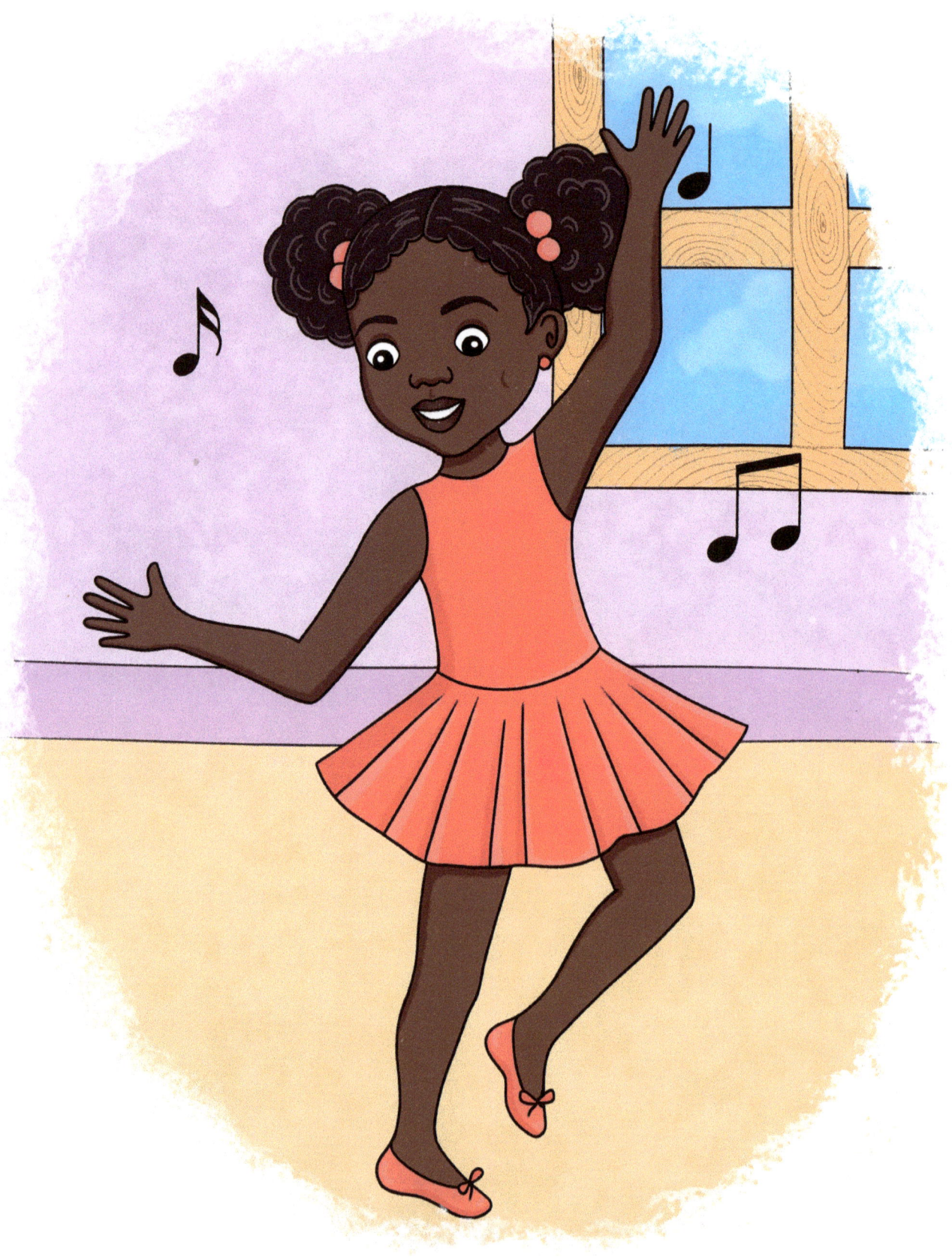

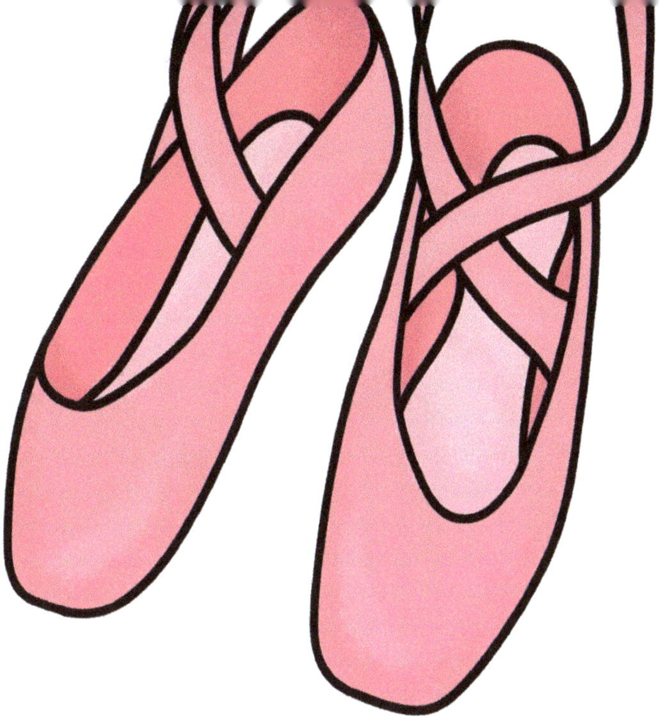

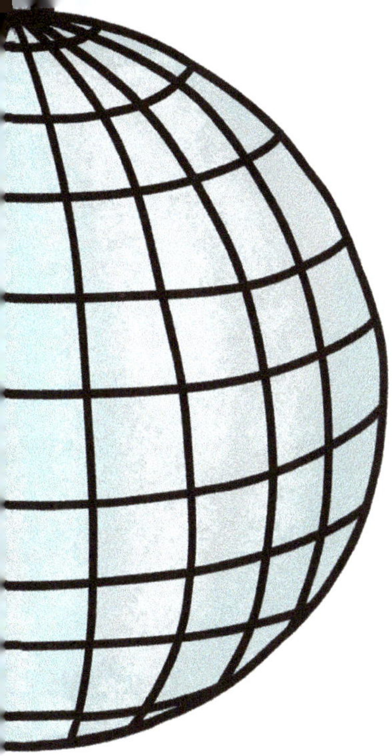

Dancing allows Serenity to express her creativity while giving her body the physical activity it needs to stay healthy. She also loves creating her own dance moves.

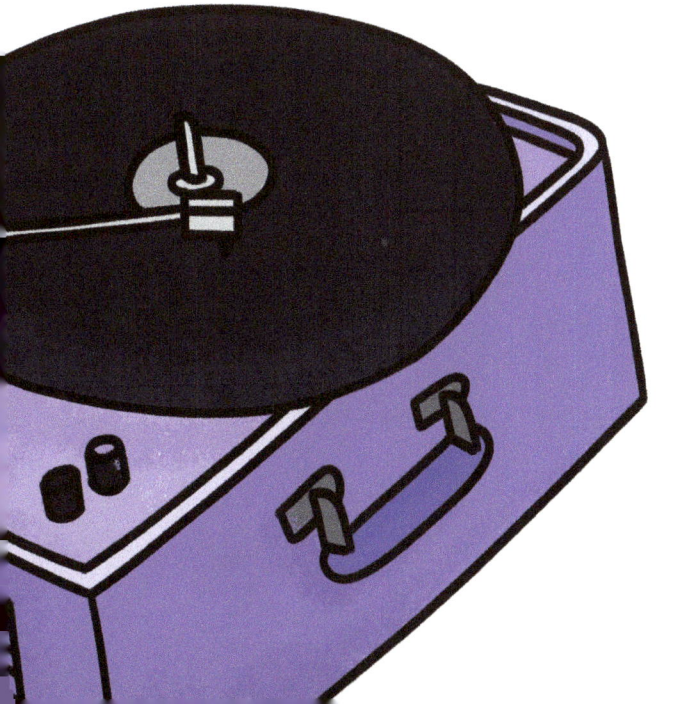
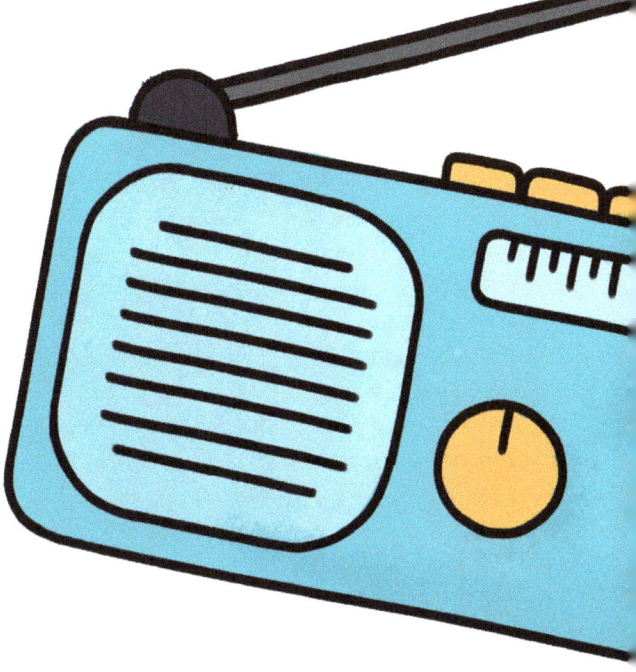

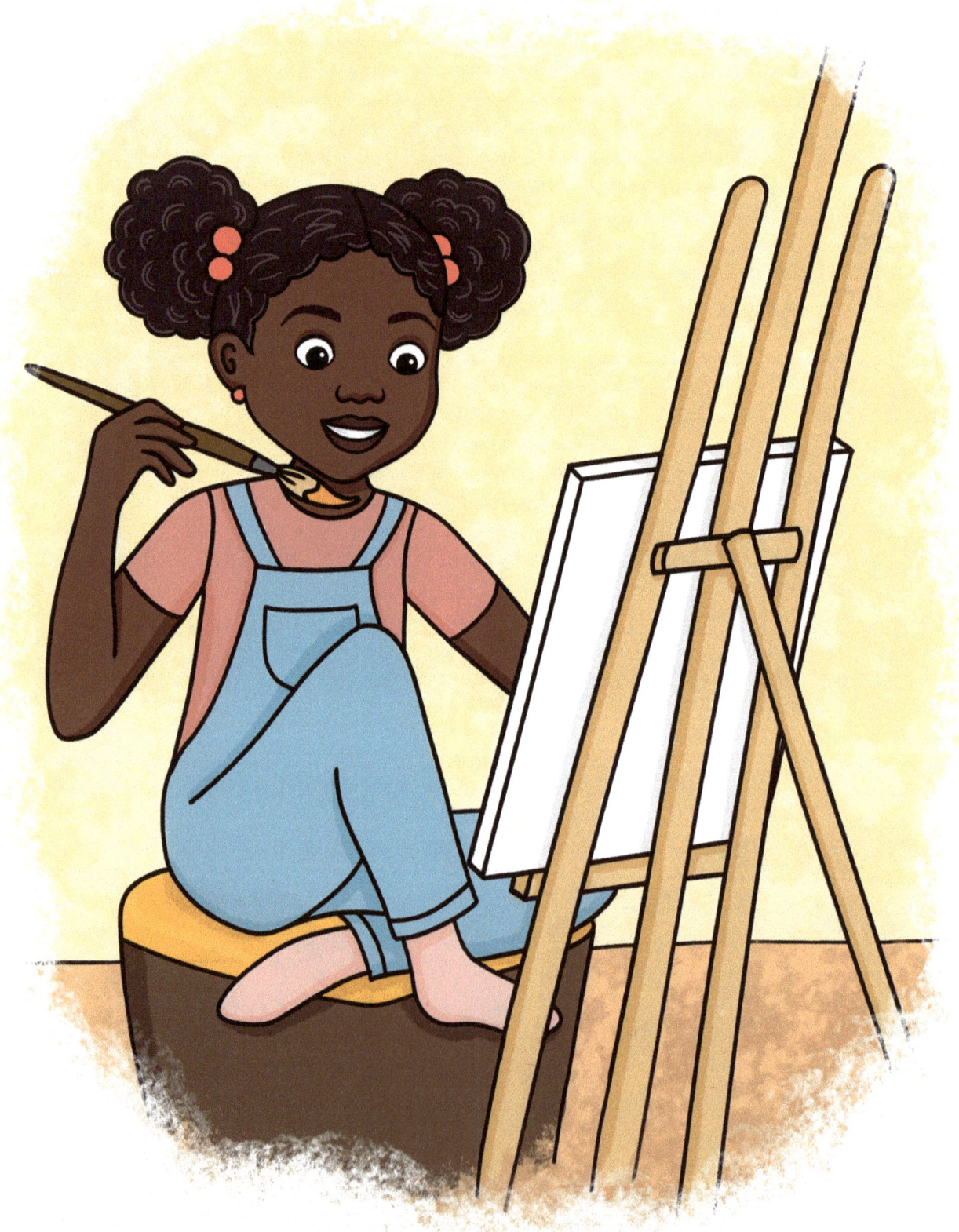

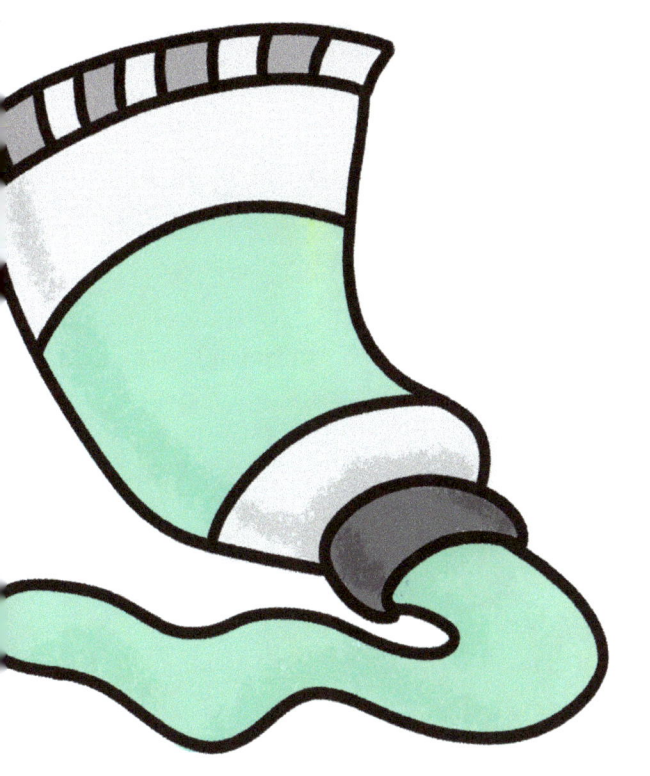

Serenity paints whatever is on her mind. She enjoys creating messy, imperfect splashes and scribbles on her canvas.

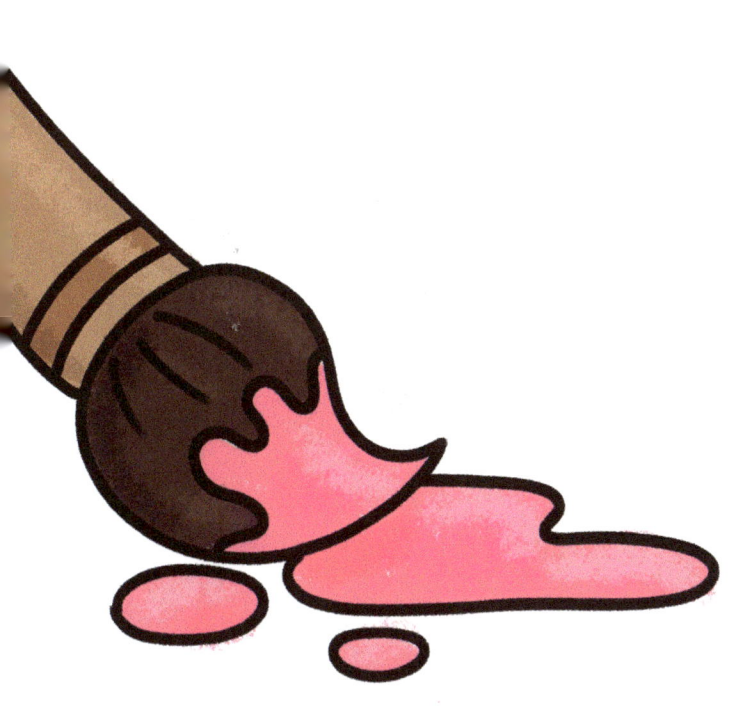
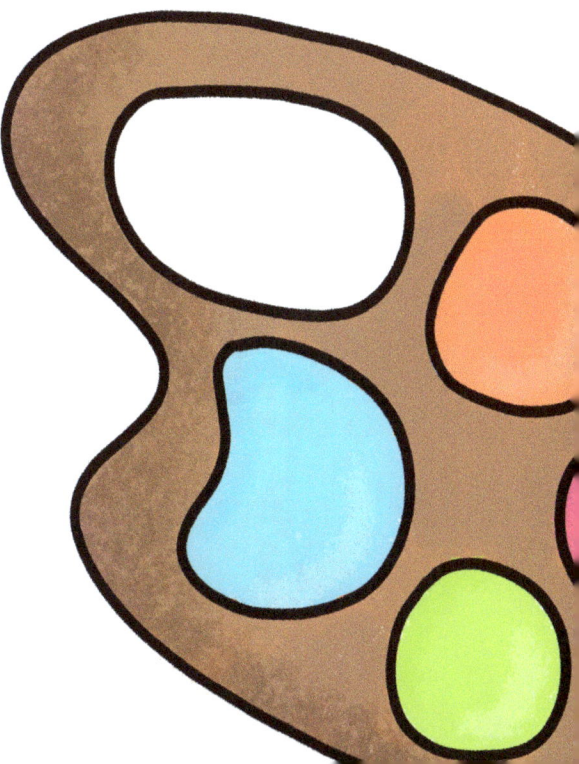

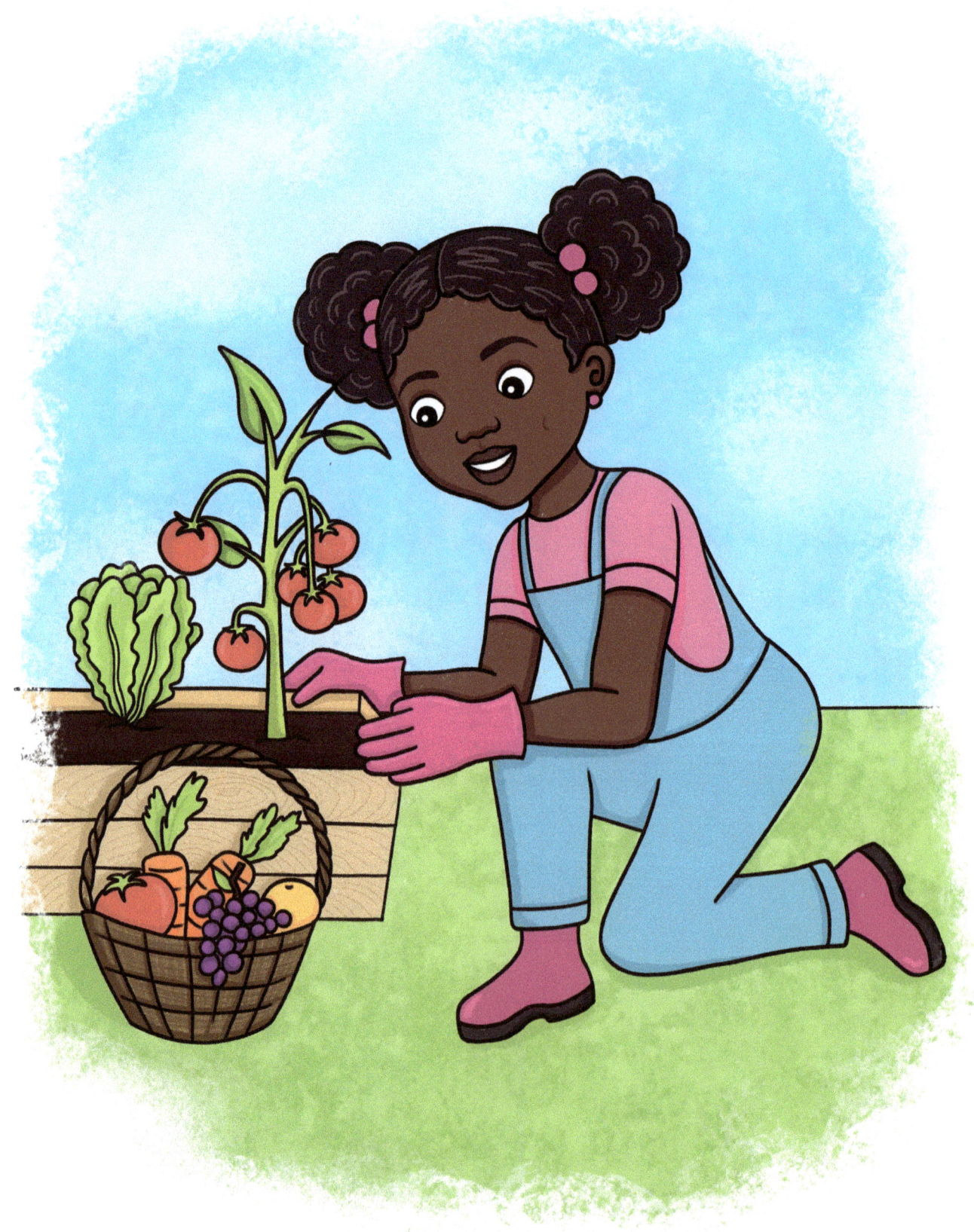

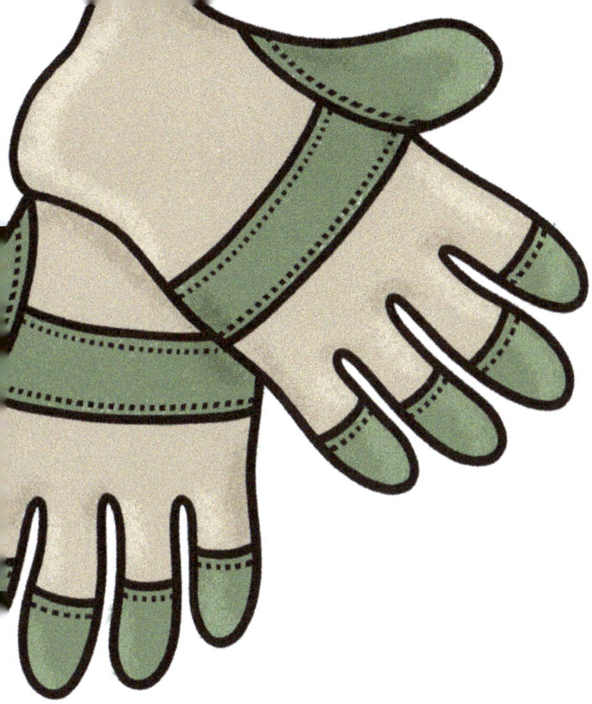

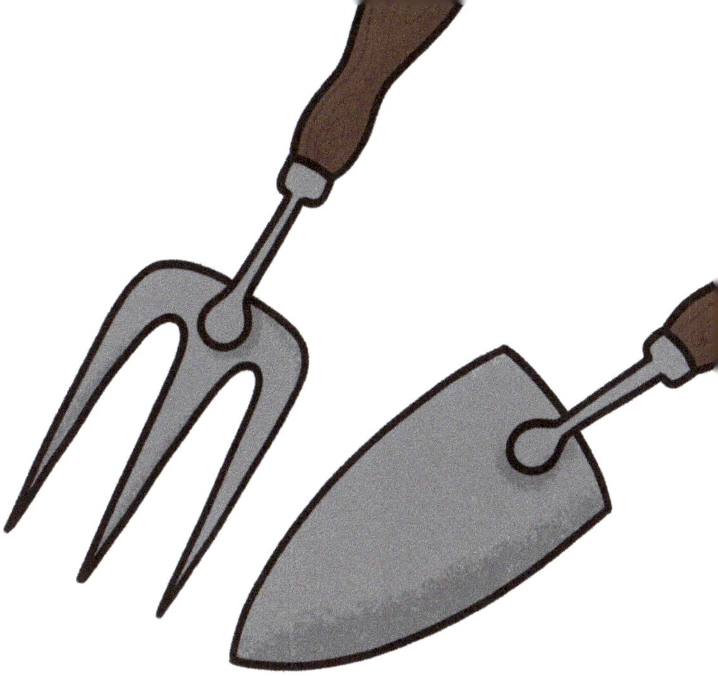

Serenity is fond of gardening for many reasons. Her number one reason is how proud it makes her to grow the freshest, tastiest produce right in her back yard that she then gets to eat!

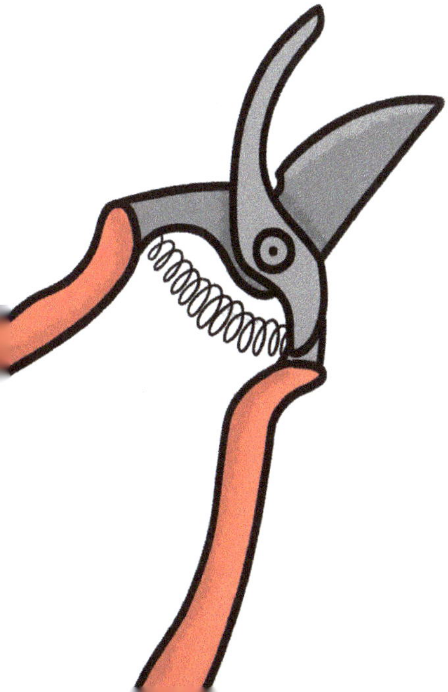

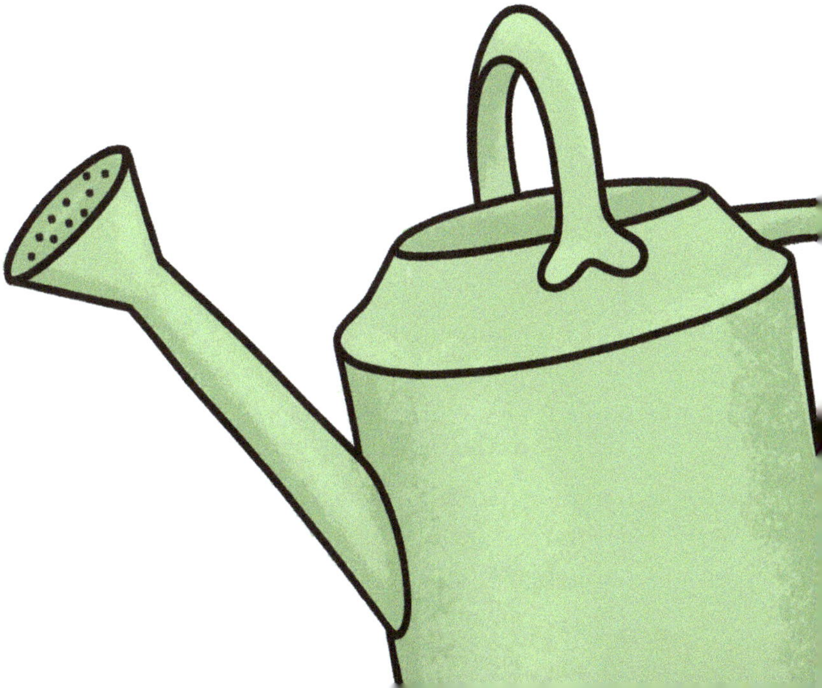

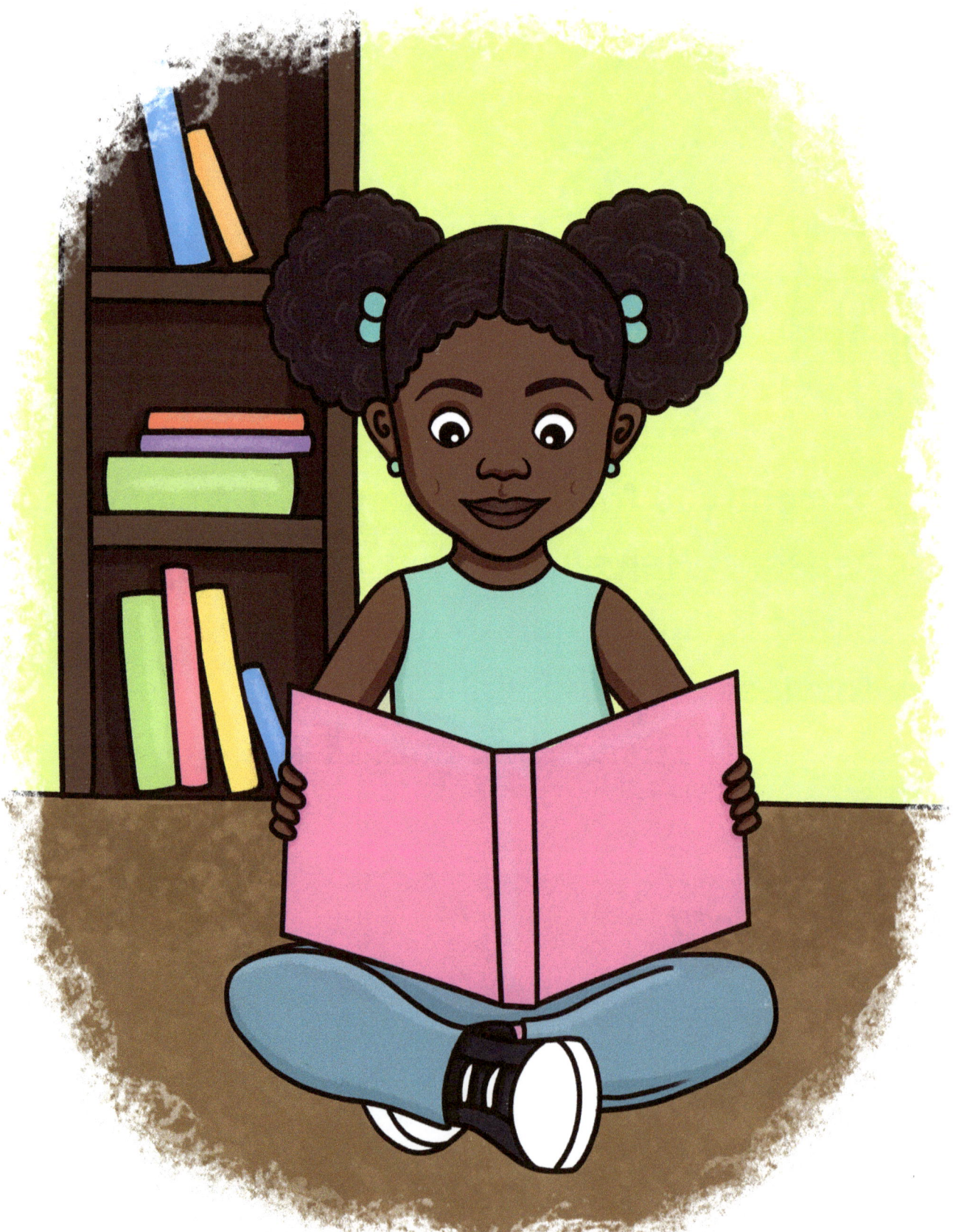

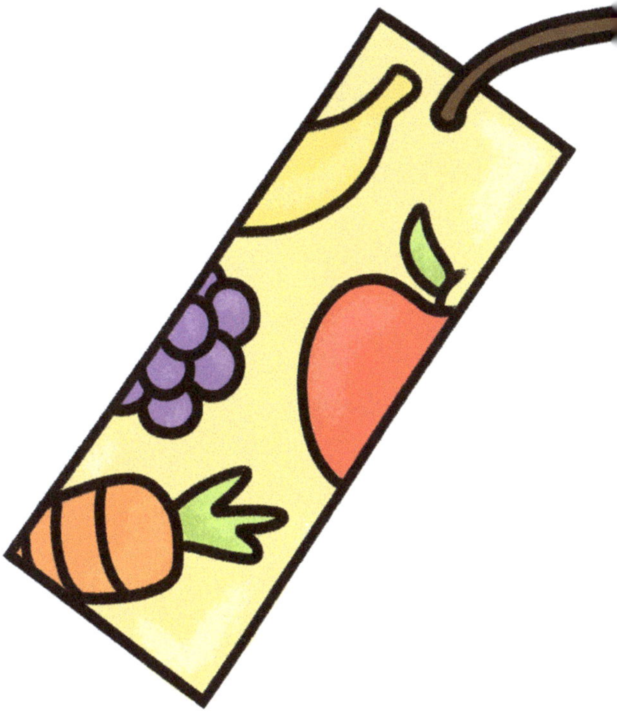

Reading has always been one of Serenity's favorite hobbies. Cuddling up with a good book keeps her laughing, learning, and a life-long fan of literature.

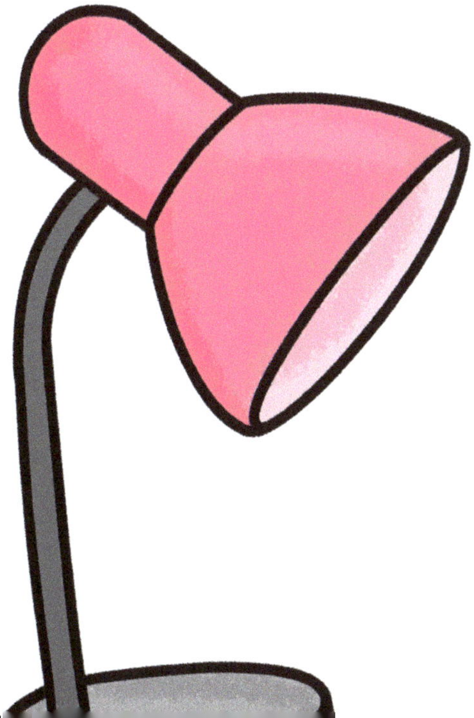

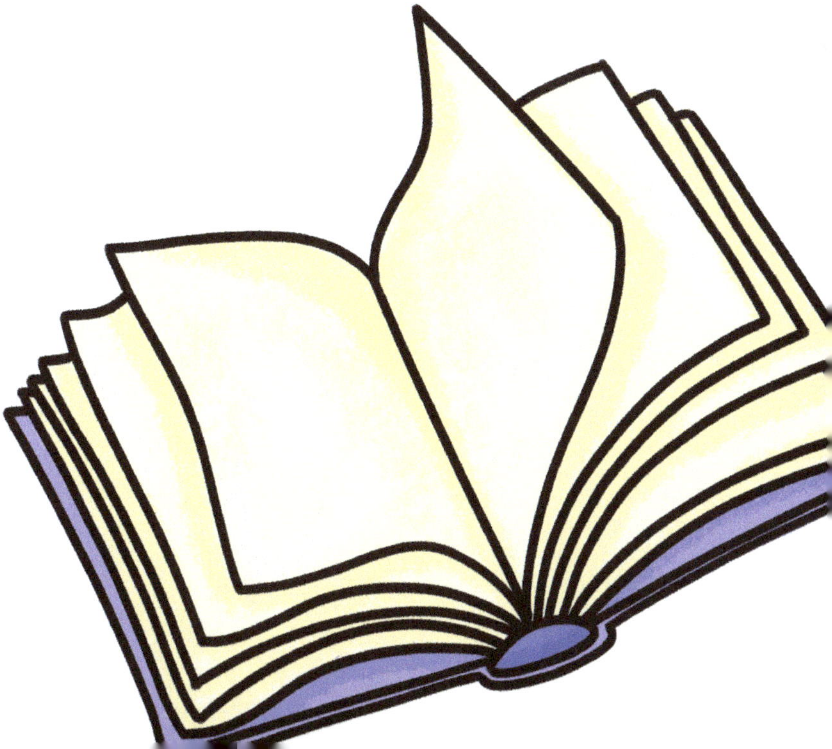

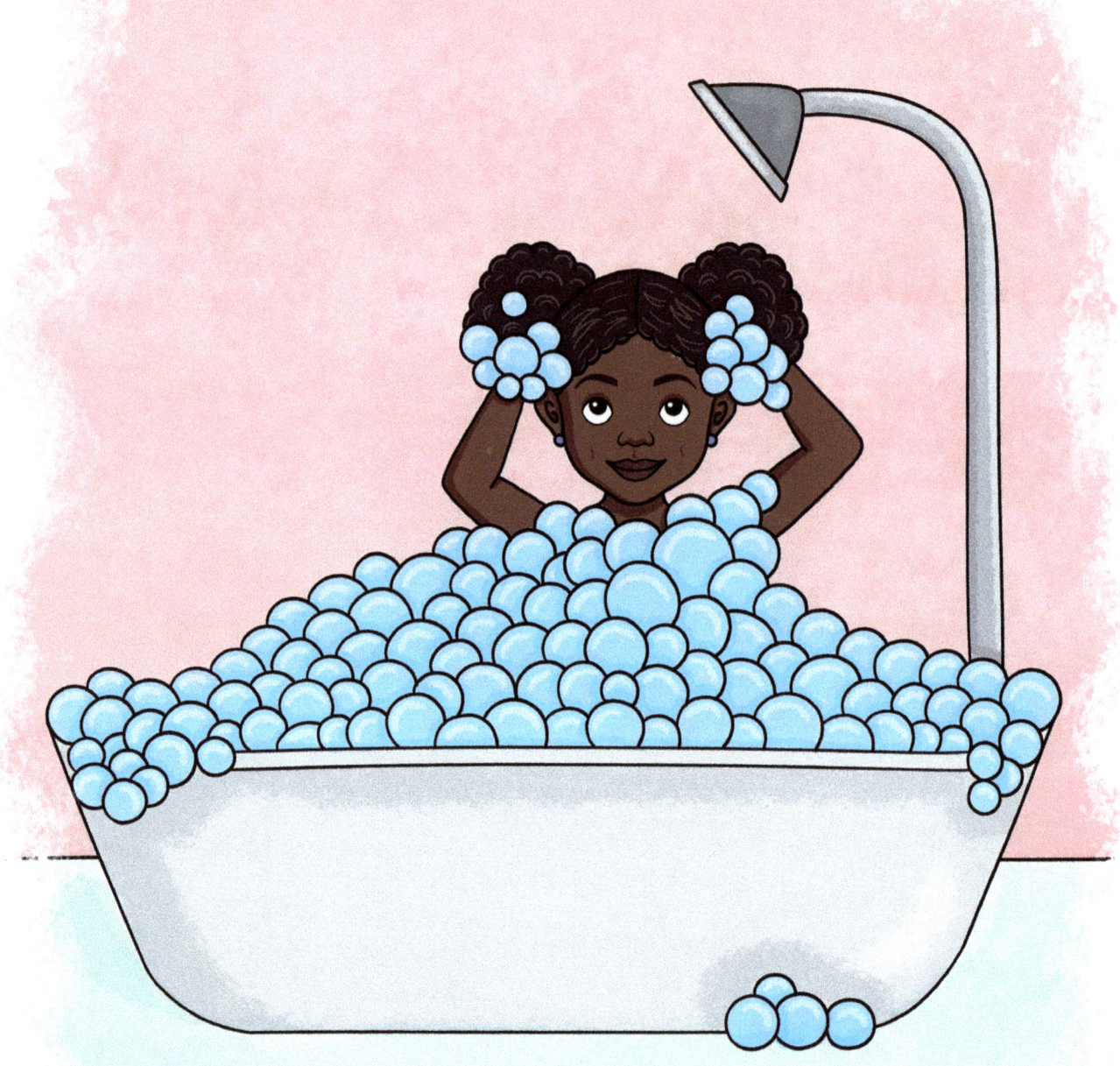

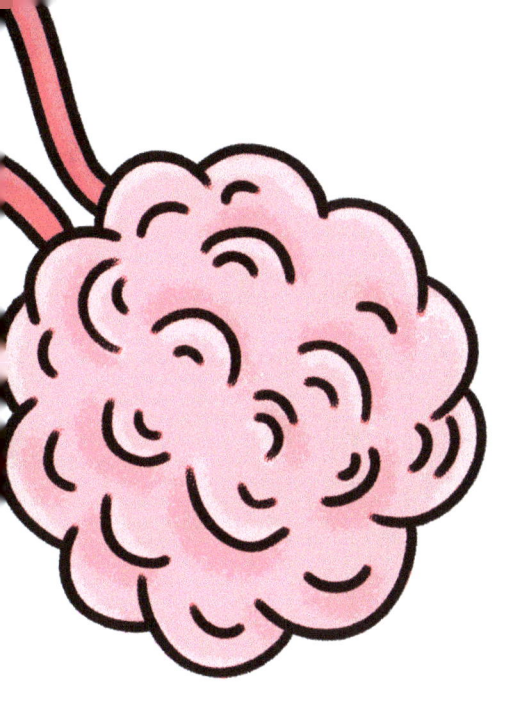
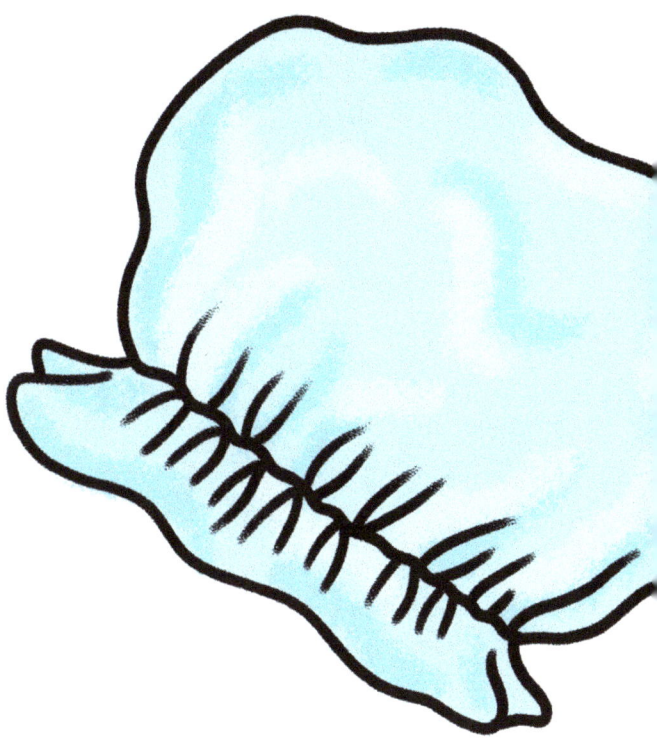

A nice warm bubble bath relaxes Serenity after a long day of learning and hobbies. Sometimes she uses a bath bomb to add relaxing smells and beautiful colors.

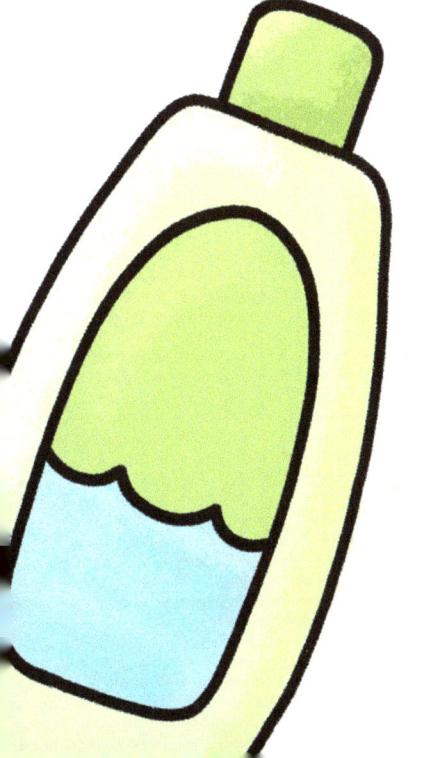
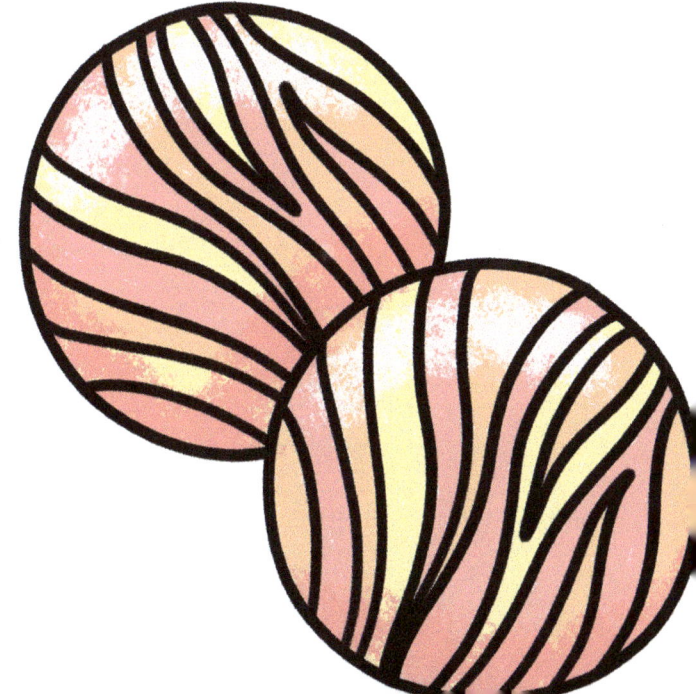

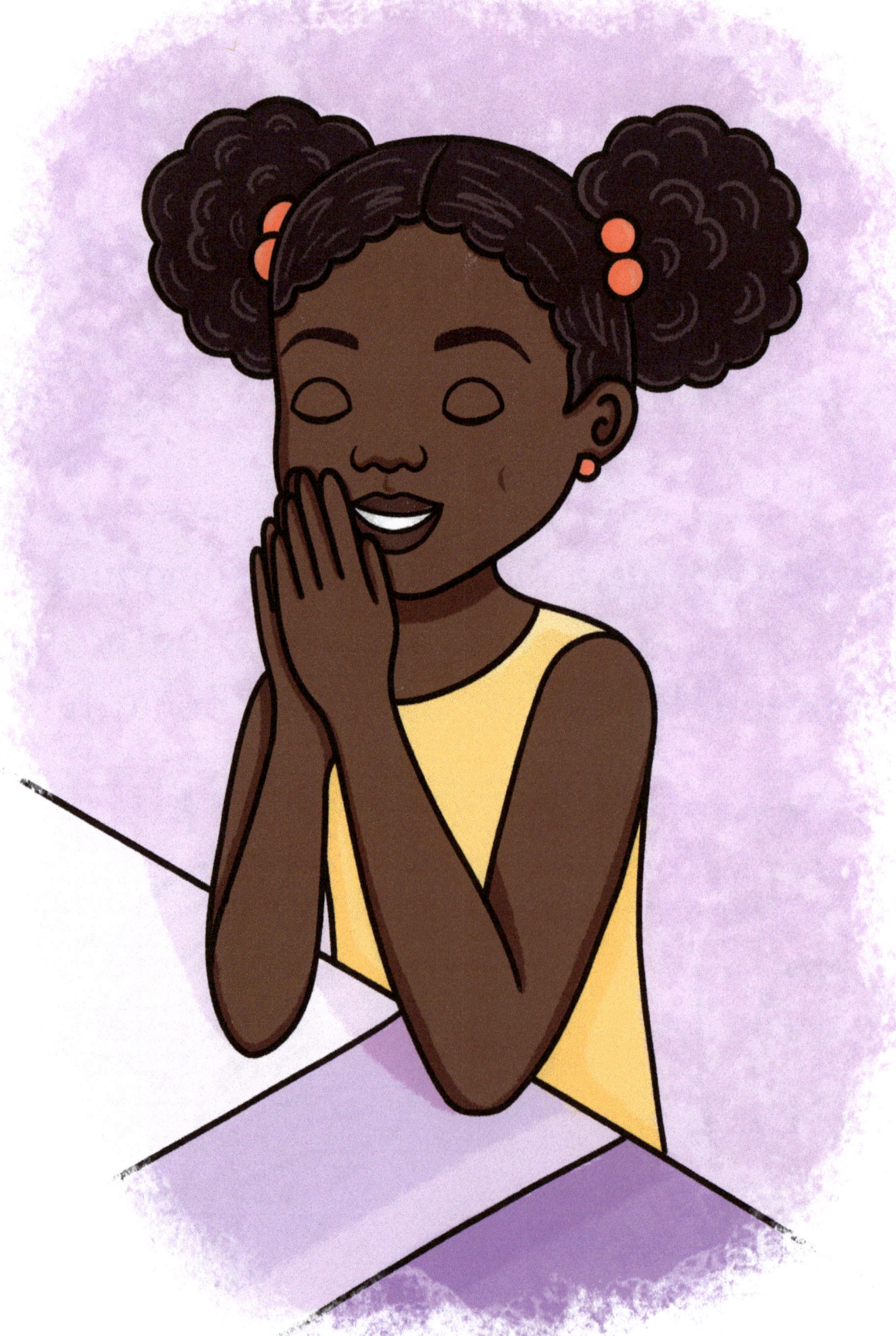

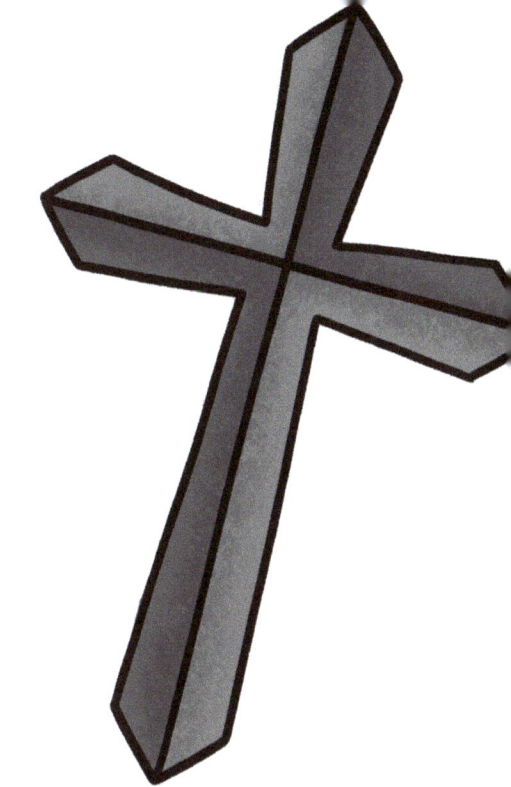

Serenity finds time every morning and evening to pray. She enjoys learning and reflecting on the word of God.

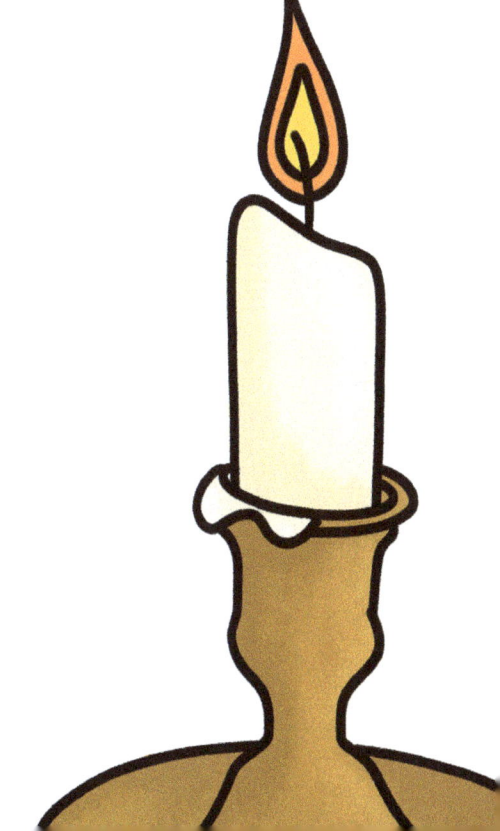

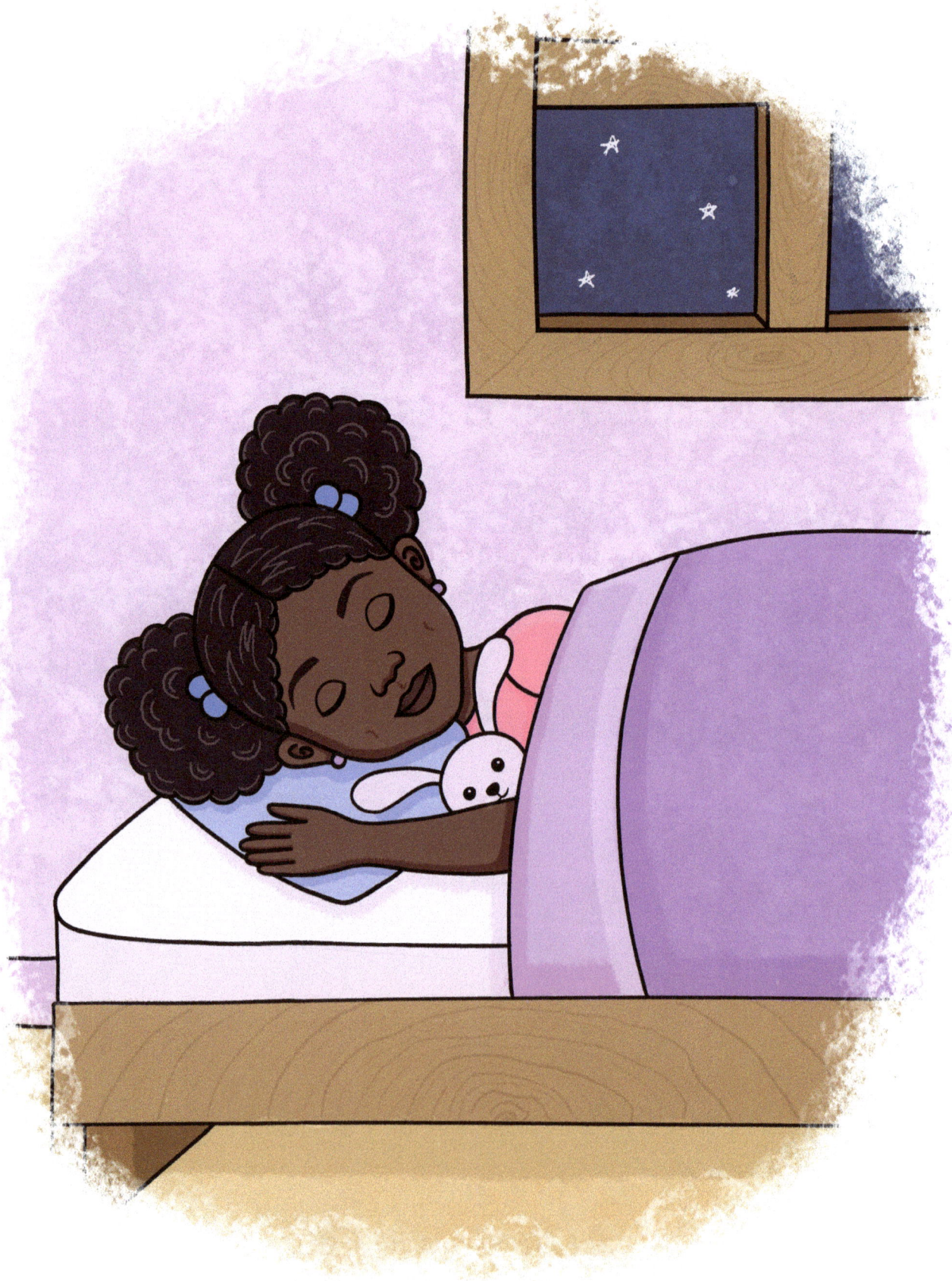

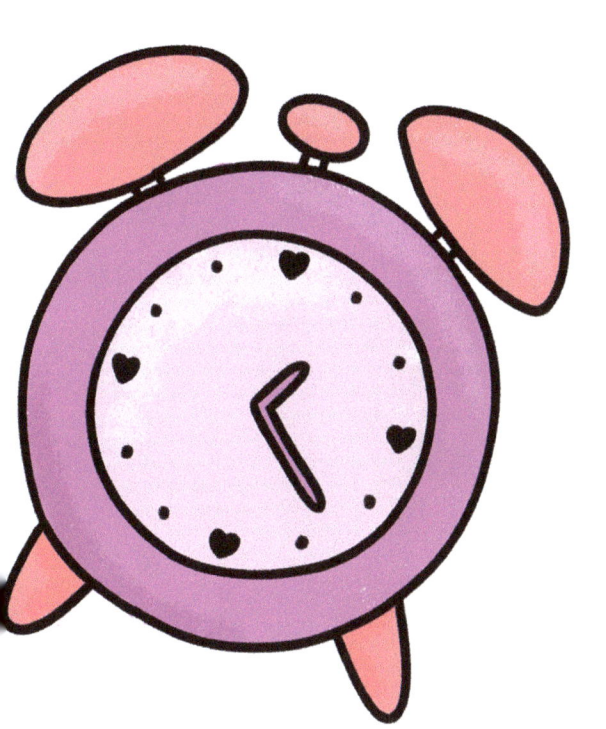
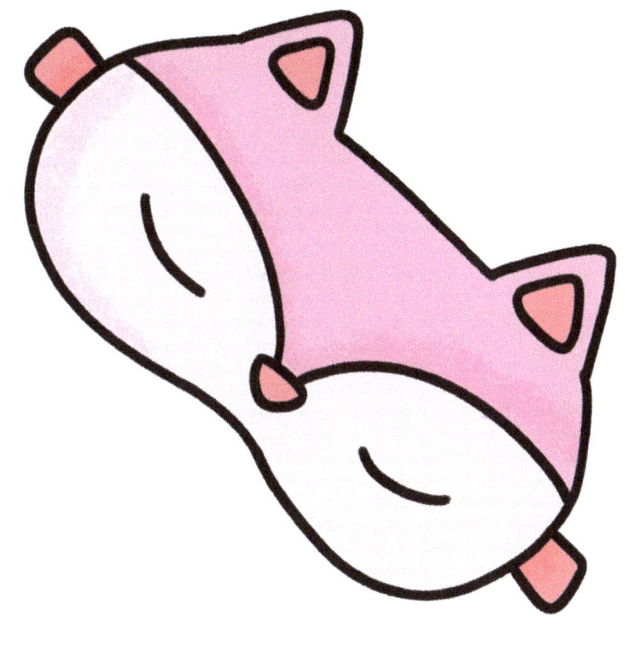

As much fun as Serenity has throughout the day, she knows the day must wind down. Sleep helps her body rest and recover for the adventures ahead.

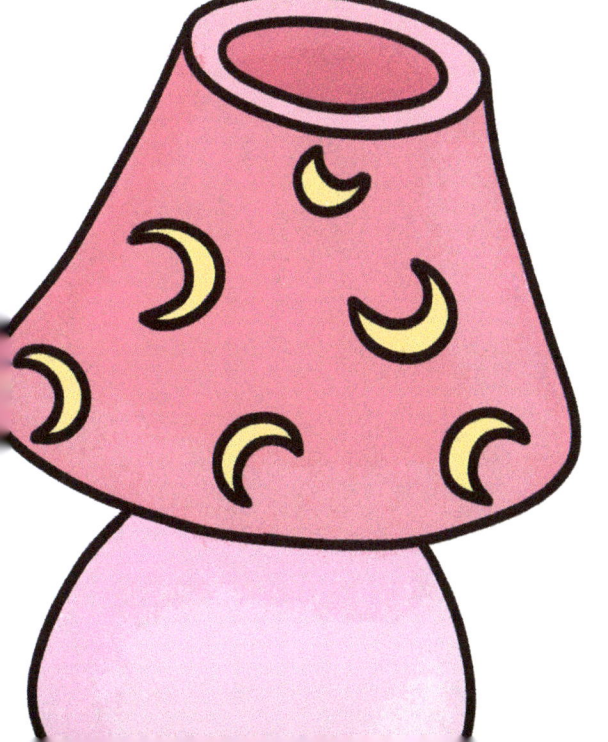
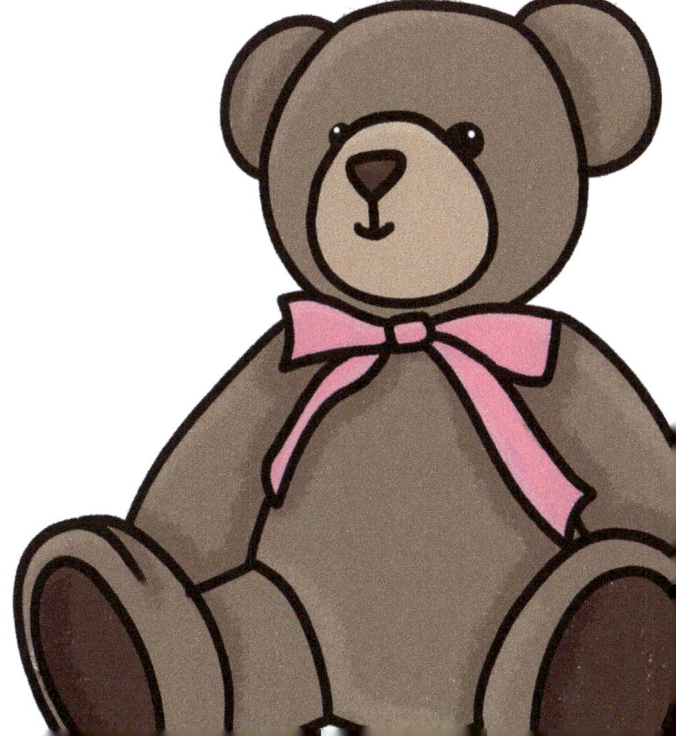

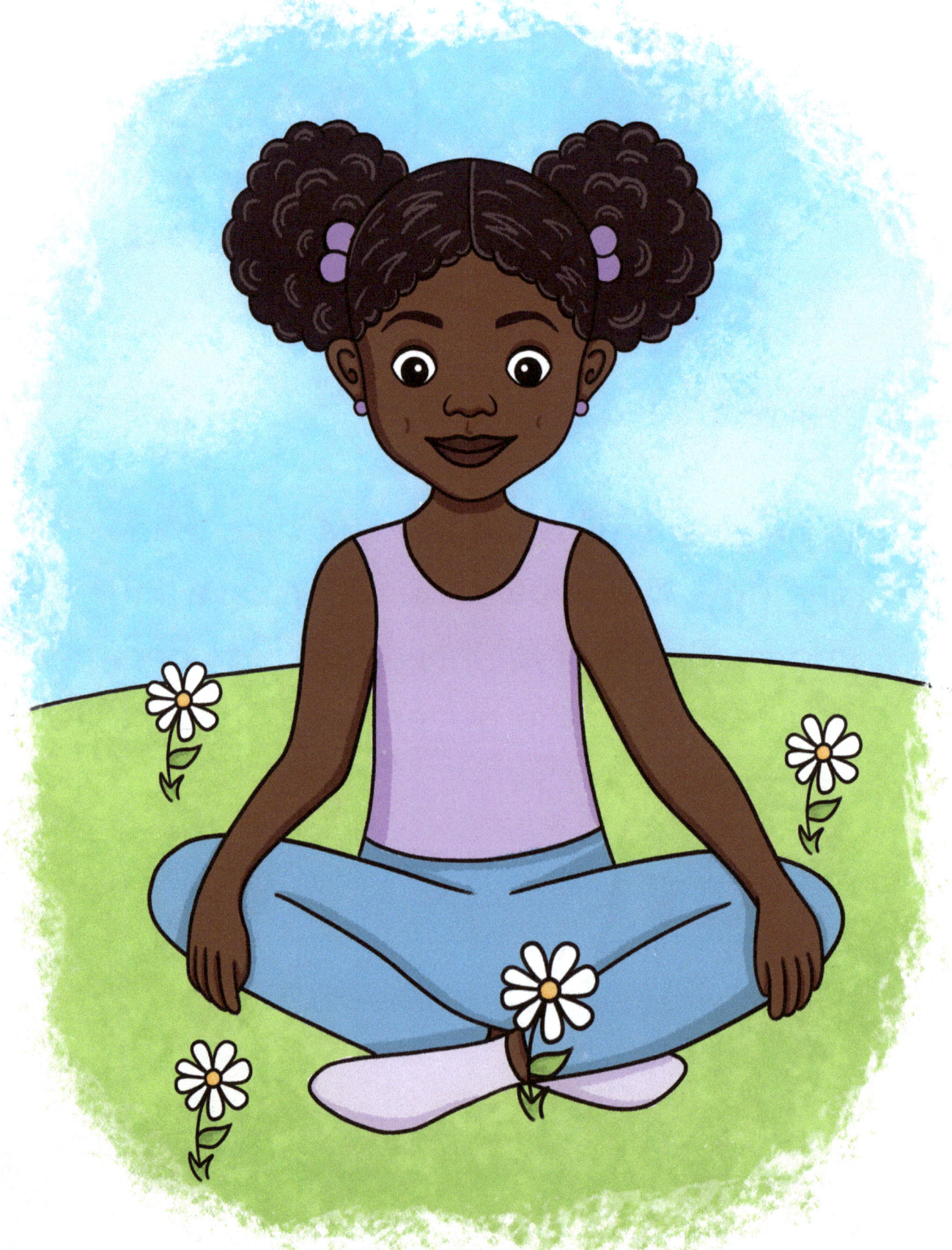

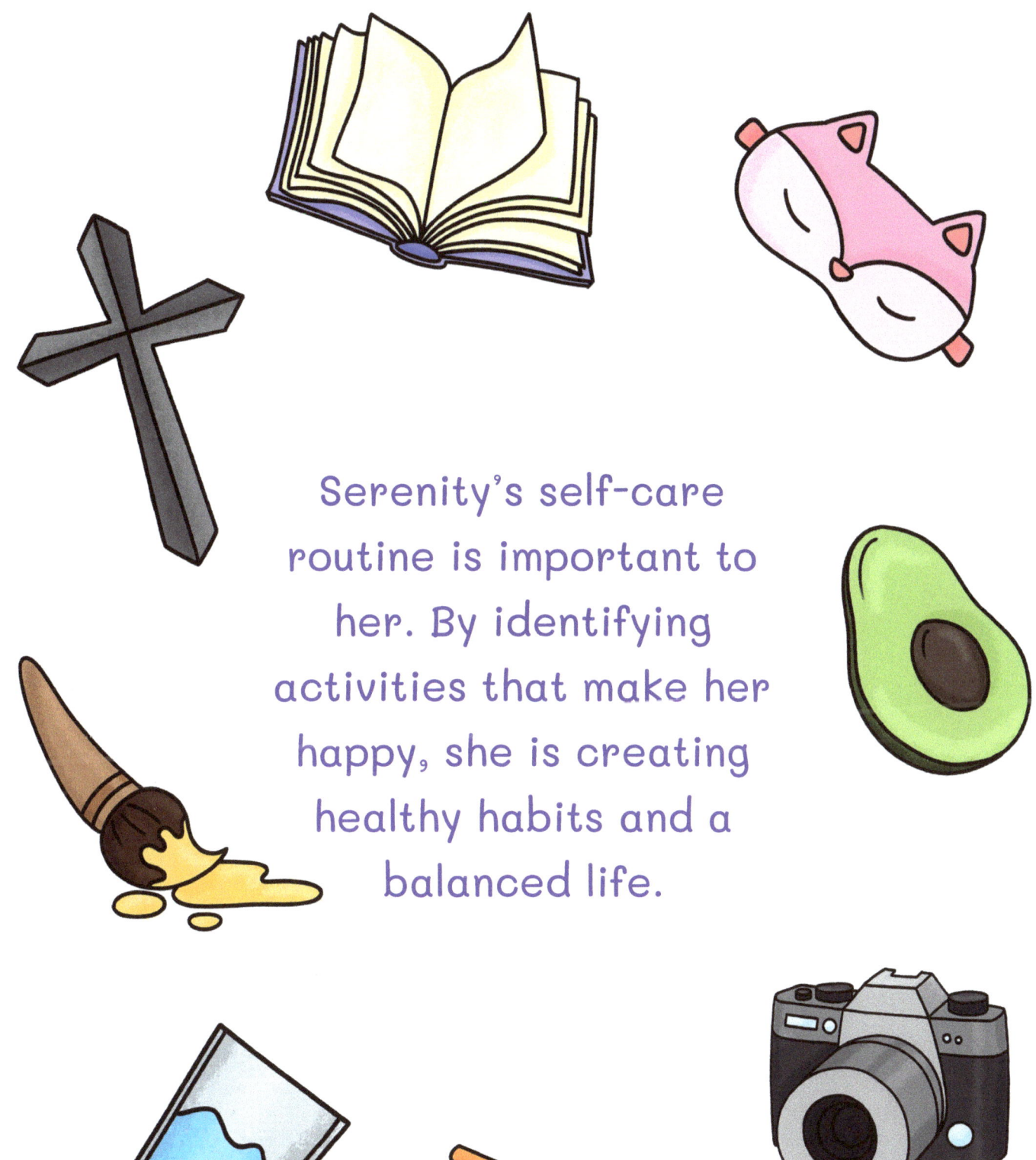

Serenity's self-care routine is important to her. By identifying activities that make her happy, she is creating healthy habits and a balanced life.

Self-Care is the best care. Take care of you and become the best version of your unique self. -DMJ

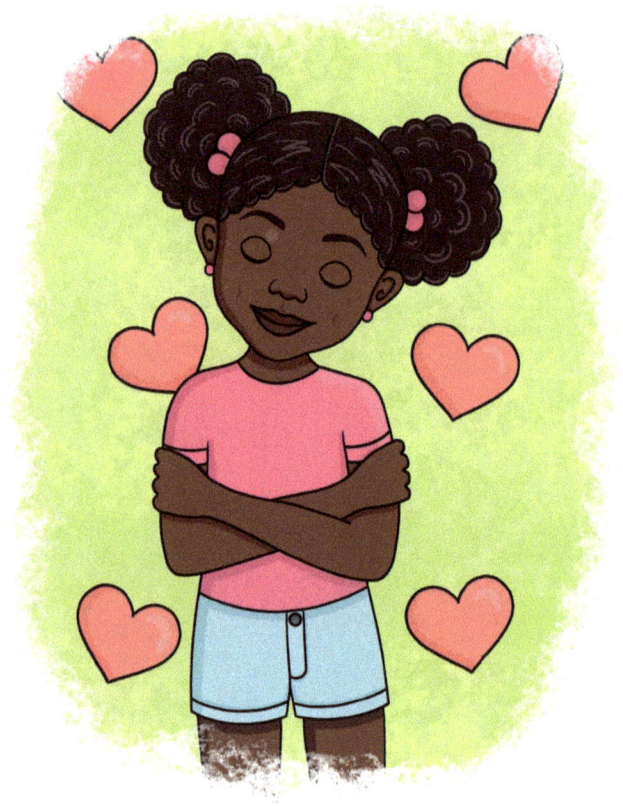

Serenity's Self-Care Routine:
A Girl's Guide to Healthy Habits
Copyright © 2022 by Hello Legendary Press LLC
Written by Danielle M. Jackson
Illustrated by Mariana Cadavid Suarez
ISBN 978-1-7361-5667-4
Library of Congress Control Number: 2022901344

All rights reserved. No part of this book may be used or reproduced in any manner whatsoever without the author's prior written permission. For information about permission to reproduce selections from this book and other work by the author, please visit www.hellolegendarypress.com/. Thank you for supporting the author's rights.

www.ingramcontent.com/pod-product-compliance
Lightning Source LLC
Chambersburg PA
CBHW051302110526
44589CB00025B/2916